The Best Way To Stop Smoking Permanently

By Andreas Michaelides

1

The Best Way To Stop Smoking Permanently.

ISBN: 978-9963-277-25-4 - Paperback

Cyprus Library.
http://www.cypruslibrary.gov.cy

Table of Contents

About the Author

Andreas was born in Athens, the city that gave birth to Democracy, in Greece, the country that taught to the world how to live, think, and have fun. He grew up on the beautiful island of Cyprus.

With both of his parent's bibliophiles (and his father a high school teacher), Andreas grew up with love and appreciation for literature. In addition to the books he borrowed from the school library, a stack of encyclopedias taught him about the world. A history lover from age 13, he devoured the memoirs of Winston Churchill and Charles de Gaul, and by age 17, he had read all of Julius Vern's books.

After serving his country for 26 months immediately after finishing high school, Andreas studied in Patra, Greece to become a computer engineer. With his Master of Computer Engineering and Informatics, he began working in the Informatics Department of the local university hospital and started reading again with a vengeance.

In 2004, Andreas authored his first book, a historical novel that has not yet seen the light of publication. Leaving it unpublished made him feel like a failure, but a lot has changed since then. Eleven years later, he has successfully quit smoking and has been smoke-free for the past six years. He has also started running again and managed to lose 26 kg (57 lbs).

Andreas has run three marathons, as well as many half-marathons and other shorter races. His love for running is what renewed him and actually saved his life.

Multiple medical problems pushed Andreas to research and experiment with a plant-based diet; since 2013 he is following a whole plant-based diet.

In addition to running, Andreas enjoys hiking, cycling, playing basketball, camping, photography, and going out with friends and family and having fun.

You can find and follow Andreas at:

Blog: www.thirsty4health.com
Facebook: https://www.facebook.com/thirsty4health/
Twitter: https://twitter.com/thirsty4health
Google+: https://plus.google.com/u/0/101942950035350104158
Linkedin: https://www.linkedin.com/in/andreas-michaelides-695351111/
Pinterest: https://www.pinterest.com/thirsty4health/
Instagram: https://www.instagram.com/thirsty4health/

Chapter 1
My Quit Smoking Story

Smoking, A Curse!

As I mentioned in my first book, *Thirsty for Health*, I had an ulcer in my stomach and my duodenum. The ulcer was caused by my junk food diet, including the consumption of caffeinated sodas and coffee, which are two highly acidic substances once they have metabolized. Smoking was another contributing factor, as it destroys the inner protective layer of your stomach that would otherwise protect you from the acidity of the hydrochloric acid secreted by the stomach.

Growing up, I would watch my father smoke with a vengeance. My mother, my siblings, and I were second-hand smokers because we lived in the same house as my dad.

Second-hand smoke comes from two sources: the end of a burning cigarette and the exhaled smoke of a smoker.

I don't remember my father smoking when we were in the same room together, but that doesn't necessarily mean it didn't happen. My mother would pester him to stop, as she would always tell us "No" in a motherly tone while waving her index finger towards my siblings and me. She never wanted us to smoke and said that our father was naughty for doing so.

Second-hand smoking is as deadly as being an actual smoker. Cigarette smoke is a carcinogen that can increase your risk of lung cancer.

Shortness of breath, wheezing, chronic cough, increased mucus, trouble controlling asthma, lung cancer, lung infections and pneumonia are also caused by being a smoker or inhaling second-hand smoke.

One good thing that Cyprus got out of becoming a member of the EU (European Union) was that the government had to apply some rules, laws, and regulations, one of which was the ban on cigarette smoking in public areas. The banning of cigarette smoking in public decreased the incidence of second-hand smoking tremendously.

Before this law was enacted, people had to endure the disgusting smoke of those sitting next to them, including a lot of places lacking proper ventilation. However, most locations now have areas distinctly dividing smokers and non-smokers, which will give non-smokers more freedom and make people efforts who want to stop smoking easier. Having a smoke-free social life after you quit smoking is an excellent form of psychological support.

When I was in high school, our theology teacher assigned us to a project, which was to write something that we would never do in our life. I wrote about smoking, and it turned out to be a decent assignment; I think I got 17 out of 20 points. I was very much convinced that I would never smoke because I had done my homework and I knew the harm smoking cigarettes cause to the body. Why would anyone intentionally start a "habit" that would only destroy his or her health? I had the knowledge that smoking causes cancer, heart disease, stroke, and lung diseases (including chronic airway obstruction, emphysema, and bronchitis).

On average, tobacco smokers die 10 years earlier than non-smokers; every cigarette smoked reduces one's life expectancy by 11 minutes. Furthermore, a single cigarette contains over 4,800 chemicals, 69 of which are known to be carcinogenic, meaning they cause cancer.

These were good, solid facts, but I didn't have the photos of lung cancer to see it and relate to it; that would help me by shocking me enough that I would never have begun smoking. But back in 1990, the Internet did not exist in Cyprus, and the only way I could have found a photo like that was in medical books, which were not widely available. Similarly, seeing a human heart damaged severely by nicotine would also have been a reminder of the awful thing that would happen to me if I started smoking.

I only acquired sterile written information, which has a much lesser impact than an image of what smoking can do to you. From my experience (as well as from reading and talking with other people), I've found that you can show smokers a ton of gruesome photos and scary facts about smoking, but they will not attempt a change until they are ready to.

I used to believe that a non-smoker should still present smokers with scary facts about smoking. In my first book, Thirsty for Health, I wrote that it could help them even if they don't see it as help at that particular moment but as an annoyance. I also wrote that it could help to bring them closer to that moment of being ready to change. I also wrote that I personally found it annoying when people would inform me of how bad smoking is (back when I smoked), but I now know that subconsciously, it helped me to reach my ready-to-change moment sooner.

After more researching and soul searching, I discovered and realized that a smoker, in reality, is *a legalized drug addict* and no matter how many gruesome pictures of a lung with cancer or scary movies or pictures are presented, they will not stop smoking because they are drug addicts. Telling a smoker that he will get that and that by smoking is like knocking on a deaf man's door. That's not the way to proceed.

I remember seeing a TV interview when I was still a high school student of the actor Yul Brynner, who died from lung cancer. You could see the remorse in his pale face from being a smoker for so many years. He was asking people not to smoke, and it made an impact on me because I liked Yul Brynner and his movies—he was, and still is, one of my favorite actors.

I remember that in my school assignment, I drew a small drawing showing a cigarette with a cobra emerging from the smoking end of it, sticking its forked tongue out. This TV interview engaged more senses than just my eyesight; it engaged my hearing also, the tone of his voice coupled with his weak gestures and the agony shown through his facial movements. It was an excellent educational tool that had the impact that I mentioned earlier, but alas, it was not enough to keep me away from smoking when the crucial moment knocked on my door.

This link is the interview that I watched so many years ago:

https://www.youtube.com/watch?v=cS3dd-OhsP4 (if the link is broken, then you can always search for it on Google or YouTube using the keywords "Yul Brynner cancer advertisement, " and you will find it).

That was when I was 17. At that time, my father was a heavy smoker; he was 43, and he had been smoking since he was 19, he picked up smoking when he went to serve his military service.

I swore to myself that I would never smoke. It was the only thing I did not like about my father, and I couldn't do anything to get my dad to stop back then.

Six months after that assignment, I finished high school. Turks invaded Cyprus in 1974—killing, raping and making refugees about 200,000 people in their own island, and until today, illegally occupy the north part of Cyprus. Because of this illegal occupation, all able males fit for military duty are required to enlist in the army after they finish high school to provide the Republic of Cyprus with the adequate military workforce.

As a result, I joined the army to serve my nation and my country for 26 months (Service is now reduced to 14 months). I am proud of my service. I learned a lot, and the army made me tougher and smarter. The army is a different society, with quick, down-to-earth lessons in reality and the hardships of life.

After some unfortunate events in my second year in the military, I started smoking in a moment of weakness. The irony was that I started smoking the same brand my father had begun smoking when he was in the army—talk about subliminal emotional messages.

I was so stupid for starting. I would cough and get dizzy every time I inhaled cigarette smoke, but for some twisted, mindless reason, I would continue to smoke until the coughing went away and the light-headed feelings were replaced by the addition of euphoria-inducing nicotine.

Like one of my cousins told me in one of our many conversations about smoking if the tobacco industries found a way to make a cigarette that would have the effect of the smoke and deliver nicotine to the brain without putting tar in the lungs, then everyone would smoke. Without knowing it, my cousin had somehow prophesied the introduction of electronic cigarettes, which, by the way, is not innocent as many people think; it's just as deadly as a regular cigarette.

Whenever I would go home on leave from the army, I would not smoke in front of my mother because I didn't want to make her sad, but my mom is no fool: she could smell my breath, and my clothes were also saturated in cigarette smoke. The cigarettes I was smoking at that point had left a yellow coating on my fingernails and my fingers of my right hand; and my teeth were a bit yellow, too. But she didn't say anything. I now wish that she had said something back then because maybe I would have stopped out of shame or not wanting to disappoint her.

So, to all mothers out there, if you know your kids smoke, confront them about it. You might get through to them or you might not, but at least you might help them to reach their realization moment much sooner.

After serving in the army, I studied at school. I got a seat on the Department of Computer Engineering and Informatics at Patra University, which was my first choice. I was very proud of myself for achieving that.

I remember I was serving the first two months of my army service (I was still in training camp) when I called my father.

After waiting for an hour to use the phone (there were no mobile phones back then) and when he told me I got the seat at the university, I jumped up, screaming from the bottom of my throat from excitement and happiness.

I remember one of the guys teased me by asking, "Are you going to be an astronaut?" But I was so happy that I just ignored the comment—and yes, I was an astronaut that moment, because I was flying with the stars; I wasn't on the ground for the next few seconds. It was one of the few amazing and memorable moments of my life, and we don't get many of those, so cherish them and live them intensely when you experience one.

When I was studying and working in Greece, smoking became part of my life. I forgot about all the bad things I knew it would do to me; I was lulled into a kind of false nirvana, which I was not aware of.

At the start, I smoked just a few cigarettes a day. Then it became a pack a day. Then 20 cigarettes a day. Then I replaced the 20-cigarette pack with a 25-cigarette pack each day. Finally, during the last years before I stopped smoking, I was up to around 60 to 80 cigarettes daily!

I experimented with all the different brands of cigarettes until I settled on one. I also used to smoke Old Holborn, which is a brand of hand-rolled tobacco. I was so clumsy when I tried to roll the first one. It was a disaster, and that alone should have made me stop smoking that kind of cigarette, but unfortunately, I saw it as a challenge I would not walk away from.

At first, I bought a hand-held rolling machine, which did expedite the cigarette-making process, but I would also practice rolling them with my hands, because carrying around that machine, the rolling paper, the lighter, and the tobacco made my pockets too bulky.

Eventually, I became good at rolling cigarettes with only one hand. I was under the false impression that because it would take me more time to prepare the cigarettes instead of picking them up from a packet, ready to smoke, that I would smoke less—I would exercise this futile practice whenever I was trying supposedly to cut down on smoking. But I would end up sitting down on the weekends and rolling the cigarettes I would smoke for that week, and I ended up smoking, even more, cigarettes than when I was buying them by the pack.

Like the American Revolution and other revolutions around the globe, there wasn't just a single revolt, but there were multiple attempts to achieve freedom from tyranny and slavery, I had a lot of failed attempts before I could free myself from the slavery of nicotine, which I was mentally and physically addicted to.

It was early October 1996 when I had just finished exams in my second year in university. Compared with previous tests, I had done well, so I wanted to make a present for myself. I always knew deep down in my heart and my soul that smoking was killing me from the inside out, blackening my lungs and spirit. I decided to try to stop smoking.

Back then, I saw smoking as something that was necessary for me, a trusted friend that was always there for me in any situation. I am sure there are smokers out there who want to stop smoking but feel like I did back then when I was still a student.

My First Attempt at Stopping Smoking

I wasn't exactly mentally ready yet to be able to stop; my mindset was not fully prepared to face the physiological and emotional steps to becoming a non-smoker. Becoming a non-smoker is a dramatic lifestyle change.

I asked other people who had supposedly successfully stopped smoking, and one of them suggested I try the nicotine replacement patch, which provides a source of nicotine that reduces the withdrawal symptoms in someone who stops smoking.

I went to the pharmacy where a friend of mine worked and asked him for nicotine patches. He was a bit surprised for two reasons: first, the only time he would see me there was when I was buying condoms, and secondly, he couldn't believe that I would stop smoking. We started talking, and he asked me how many cigarettes I smoked a day, which brand I smoked, and how many milligrams of nicotine the cigarettes contained.

I asked him why all the questions, and he said my answers were crucial to determine the strength of the patch and the length of time to be used.

He told me to apply the patch to a clean, hairless, dry area on my upper arm; I should only use one every 24 hours unless I wanted to overdose and leave this planet. Despite nicotine's high toxicity, a person cannot overdose on nicotine just by smoking. Overdose, however, can happen if a person uses too many nicotine patches or chews too much nicotine gum. He also told me to replace the piece patch at a given moment and that I could wear it even during taking a shower, which I thought was cool because I could still get my fix while water was dropping on me, something I couldn't do while smoking a cigarette.

Finally, he showed me how to apply the patch. He mentioned that in two weeks time, I should come back to get a patch with a smaller dose, gradually decreasing the dose with the ultimate goal to completely remove it from my system.

I went home and put the nicotine patches packet on my handmade coffee table, which was a stack of books that I read and a piece of wood on top. I sat on the bed and stared at the pharmacy bag, wondering whether I was ready and whether I was strong enough to be victorious.

It was around 6 p.m. when I applied my first patch. I had to remember to change the old with the new same time daily so I wouldn't get any withdrawal symptoms.

The first two days were okay. It seemed that I didn't have the urge to smoke, maybe because I stayed home and did household chores, read a book, and had pretty good control over my actions.

The third day, I had to go out for a coffee, and that's when it hit me. I wanted to smoke so badly. I always smoked while having my coffee, plus all my friends were smoking. Seeing all the automatic mouth and hand gestures urged me to pick up a cigarette and light it, put it in my mouth and inhale a long-lasting puff and then hold it for a few seconds in my lungs before exhaling the dark smoke of sin into the air.

But I managed to withstand the urge, even after all the teasing from my friends, who didn't want me to stop smoking. (If you want to quit smoking, from personal experience, you need to temporarily stop hanging around people that smoke, at least first two to three weeks).

The fourth day was doomsday. I broke down when I and "the gang" went out to a club with loud music, dancing, and drinking. I had never been a heavy alcohol drinker, but I would always smoke when having a beer or my very rare whiskey, and that's when I gave in. I lit a cigarette, and as you smokers know, it only needs to be one to become a smoker, so my first try at stopping was a failure; the nicotine patch didn't work for me.

Apply the patch in different spots and not on top of the previously used space. I only used the patch for four days, but it gave me a rush because I didn't use another spot. (I was too lazy to shave the hair on my arm to make space for other patches. What can I say? I like my hair.)

I didn't experience any of the common side effects, maybe because I used it for only four days.

I guessed when he didn't see me after two weeks; the pharmacy guy would assume he was right about me. Of course, he saw me again, as I had to buy condoms anyway.

Electronic Cigarettes

Back then, electronic cigarettes were not available in Greece, so I didn't have the pleasure of trying that to stop smoking. I have read a lot of good reviews, and it seems to be a healthier alternative than smoking real cigarettes, but they do still have deadly effects because of the nicotine. Of course, there is also the side effect of coughing up tar, which happens whether you switch to e-cigarettes or stop entirely; it's because your body is trying to get rid of the tar in your lungs because you're no longer adding to the problem by smoking cigarettes made by tobacco leafs.

While e-cigarettes are considered healthier because they have no tar, they still have nicotine, so if you switch to e-cigarettes, you will remain an addict. I think if e-cigs had been available when I was attempting to stop, I would be smoking them today.

Quitting Smoking: Second Attempt

My second attempt at stopping smoking was also a disaster. After the nicotine patch failure, I decided to stop smoking cold turkey. I ceased buying cigarettes, threw away all of my matches and lighters, and gave away all of my ashtrays. I was determined to get rid myself of this culprit finally.

I lasted for a week, which was fantastic, especially considering I had chosen the worst week of my life to stop smoking: final exams week. On the sixth day of that week, I started crying for no reason; I would just start to cry while doing anything, even eating, and suddenly tears would run down my face. I didn't know what was happening to me. I called my parents and told them that I couldn't seem to stop crying, and after a little benevolent interrogation, I mentioned to them that in addition to dealing with my final exams, I had also decided to quit.

They told me (to be fair I don't remember if it was mom dad or both of them) to start smoking again because that was probably the cause of my sudden crying bouts. Their advice was a bit of a shock to me because I had expected a more supportive attitude towards my decision to stop smoking—the last thing I had expected to hear was advice to start smoking again.

They were right, though. As soon as I started smoking again, the crying bouts stopped. I think the combined stress of the exams and stopping smoking was the cause of my crying, as I was neither physically nor emotionally ready for the challenge of such a drastic change

Quitting Smoking: Third Attempt

I like reading books a lot, which is something I inherited from my parents, who are both avid readers. Around 1998, on one of my trips to the USA, I sat on the plane next to a lady who had a book in her hand titled The Easy Way to Stop Smoking.

Curious by nature, I asked her what the book was about. She told me that the author claimed that when you finished reading this book, you would stop smoking; she also said you don't have to quit while reading it.

The thought stuck in my mind, and years after, when I returned to Cyprus and worked as a substitute teacher, I saw one of my colleagues reading the same exact book. I remembered the lady on the plane telling me about it, so I asked her where I could find a copy. My colleague gave me the name of a bookstore, and the next day, I bought one.

I read it while I had my breaks between classes, and it took me a month to finish. It is a fantastic book that methodically debunks every reason or excuse someone may have not to quit smoking, and it lets you decide whether you want to keep smoking or not.

To be honest, I did not follow all of the directions in the book (maybe that's one of the reasons it did not work with me), but it did leave an impact on me. When I finally stopped smoking, all of my previous failed attempts to quit helped me to achieve my present cigarette-free state.

In 2005, I returned to Cyprus. Of course, at the time, I was still a smoker. I would smoke in front of my mother, and with my father, we would buy cartons of cigarettes that we would smoke together, which totaled about 200 cigarettes a week on average.

I kept myself busy by working three jobs from Monday to Friday and helping my father with his farming chores over the weekends. Juggling three jobs made me feel very anxious, and whenever I got anxious or stressed, I would light a cigarette.

My Moment of Realization

I smoked until May 2009, when something changed me.

I would always wake up in the morning without being able to breathe satisfactorily; my nose would always be blocked, and I didn't have a sense of smell. My mother has beautiful roses in her garden that smell fantastic, but I couldn't detect their aroma, nor could I feel the jasmine picture that was on our front porch. Because smoking had stifled my sense of scent, I was also unable to smell food and the different flavors in it.

When I was a student in Greece, and later in life, I would get the flu very easily and very often; I would get sick at least five to six times in a year. Now, if it only took a couple of days to get well from the flu and colds, that would be no issue worth mentioning, but unfortunately, it would always take about 7 to 10 days to recover fully.

While I was ill, my nose was blocked, my chest always felt like a fat man had sat on it, and I also suffered psychologically. I was so sick that I couldn't enjoy smoking, which subconsciously informed me that I could live without it because when I was sick, I could go without smoking for 7 to 10 days, and I didn't have any cravings or urges (which I always found weird).

During that time, my body would clean out some of the ugly stuff. Altogether, I was sick for around 4 to 6 weeks each year! Me being sick often was because of the destructive effects that smoking had on my immune system and other systems.

The reason smokers get sick more frequently and more severely is because the cigarette smoke prevents the cilia (the "brooms" of the lungs) from cleaning the lungs.

Also, the lungs and the airways have more mucus, which clogs them and makes you cough; this extra mucus that cannot be removed can easily result in an infection.

Smoking destroys the lung tissue, reducing the air capacity, which means less oxygen is carried to the body, and overall, you are less protected from infection because the natural defenses that your lungs have against infection don't work as well.

I also noticed that I gained a lot of weight; I was 84 kg (185 lbs), and I am 1.74 m (5 feet 9 inches) tall. I was overweight, and I knew that when you smoke, you don't gain as much because it

17

curbs one's appetite, but there I was, a smoker who was overweight—not a very safe and healthy combination. I was a heart attack or stroke waiting to happen, and I was only 35 years old!

I was tired all of the time (my three jobs were sedentary ones, and I never had the time or motivation to exercise). I also started getting nasty acne on my chest and shoulders.

One of my three jobs was as a computer technician. One day, I got a call from a customer asking me if I had finished fixing his PC. I had, and he said because he was in a hurry, he would drive over, and I should meet him on the road and deliver his PC there.

From my place on the road is a small hill. Because I had other things on my mind, I completely forgot that I had to meet the guy, so he gave me a call while he was on the street to remind me. I answered, I apologized, and then I grabbed the PC and ran uphill to go to the road. I couldn't believe that I almost didn't make it; I was aching everywhere, my lungs were screaming for oxygen, and I couldn't catch my breath. I almost dropped the computer, and the guy thought I had a heart attack.

That's when I woke up. All of my previous knowledge about smoking, all of my previous failed attempts at stopping, and all of the experiences around smoking somehow came together like a jigsaw puzzle and woke me up, breaking the fog that had prevented my mind from seeing the road.

The next day, I had an appointment with my dermatologist about the acne on my chest. One the things he said I should do was stop smoking: I think it was the first time I heard someone telling me that, and I agreed with him without getting angry.

Coming home with my father driving, we were smoking together, and I said that I wanted to quit. To my surprise, my dad agreed with me and said, "Yes, let's stop smoking." I think we smoked our last cigarette together in the car, or maybe we finished the last pack that we had on us the next day, but what matters is that we are both smoke-free since 2009.

Remorse

The next day, my father did not buy any cartons of cigarettes. We told my mother that we would stop smoking, and I don't remember mom ever being happier in her life. By smoking in front of her, we had poisoned her with our smoke—and passive smokers have it the worst, because they only inhale all of the nasty stuff, like tar, without even having the "reward" of the nicotine.

I felt bad that I had been a smoker for 16 years and that my smoking had hurt the people around me, including people I cared about, like my mother. While teaching at a private high school, I remember my students telling me that the exercises and their tests (which I would take home to correct and grade) smelled of tobacco. At the time, I thought they were crazy or lying to me (probably because my sense of smell was dulled), but they were right, and I can see that now.

Before I stopped smoking, one very dear first cousin of mine stopped smoking years before me. I remember standing outside his door, smoking, and I asked him something related to smoking—he told me that if I respected him and also respected myself, I would never smoke in front of him. That made me angry because it hit a nerve. I knew he was right, but in a twisted, unreasonable way, I was not ready to accept it. But now I see he was right because he was in the state of mind that I am now. Now, I see other people smoking, and I see them for what they really are, drug addicts that need help.

Telling the World

I announced to my colleagues, friends, and relatives that I was no longer a smoker because I knew that if everyone knew I had stopped smoking, I would have peer pressure not to start again, which would help me to remain a non-smoker.

My father and I threw away our matches, lighters, and ashtrays; anything that reminded us of cigarettes vanished.

Stopping to smoke forever wasn't easy. I think the reasons I managed to finish once and for all were that, first, I wasn't alone. I was stopping with my father, which was good because we were supporting and helping each other. Secondly, I was mentally and emotionally ready: I wanted to stop because I finally understood what I had been doing to myself and others around me for the last 16 years (which was killing myself slowly, cigarette by cigarette, removing about eleven minutes of my life every time I finished smoking a cigarette).

On Tuesday, May 19th, 2009, I decided to quit. This decision played a major role in my life, as it was a very significant, active catalyst for my present health status. My father and I chose to get rid of the filthy addiction; thankfully, we were victorious at the end.

To any other people out there who belong to the significant percentage of individuals who quit smoking and remain non-smokers: quitting smoking is a big success for you, and you should celebrate your accomplishment every year with friends and family. Make a big thing out of it and reward yourself for remaining a non-smoker. If you think about it, you should celebrate this kind of life-changing anniversary with even more enthusiasm than your birthday, name day, or marriage. You are celebrating your anniversary of stopping smoking. You were reborn into a new, healthier, happier you; a better version of you emerged, and a new destiny awaits you.

Withdrawals

The three first weeks of stopping smoking were psychologically hell for me. The nicotine withdrawal symptoms started almost immediately after my dad, and I had our last cigarette.

I couldn't sleep well, but then again, I hadn't had a restful sleep in years. Stopping smoking wasn't the only reason for my insomnia, but it did intensify it; I could feel a big hole in my chest that was my craving for a cigarette.

I was unfocused, irritable, and I lost my temper very quickly, which is why I didn't get much work done during those days (I didn't want to scare away any customers with my bad mood). I had a constant mental itch in my head as if someone were pricking me with a needle; even today, just thinking about how it felt makes me want to scream.

I also started to eat a lot more than I used to because my appetite had increased. When I would sit in front of a computer (either installing programs or fixing something hardware related), I would usually smoke. Now, I had to do something else with my hands and my mouth instead so I would eat sandwiches, croissants, chips, and drink ice tea and non-caffeinated soda (I gave up caffeine years ago because of my stomach ulcer).

One of the little life experiences that helped me to realize that I could stop smoking and that smoking was not useful or necessary for me was my freedom from caffeine. I figured, "If I could rid myself from caffeine, then why not free myself from nicotine, too?"

I read somewhere that nicotine will leave your body by a fat percentage within three weeks of quitting. I told myself that if I can last for three weeks without smoking, then I will not have any excuse for wanting to smoke because the addictive agent will not be on my system; so that was another reason never to smoke again.

Success

I managed to get through the first three weeks. During those three weeks, I did not go out with friends. I avoided all acquaintances and relatives or situations in which I might have to see another person smoke, and I even stayed away from the TV in case I saw a movie where people would be smoking.

The first three weeks are very crucial to your success as a non-smoker; you need to become a little hermit (as social life is concerned) for a while before you go outside and into the world. For other people, it might be a little more or a little less than three weeks, but you will need that period to build your confidence, to be able to admit to yourself and convince yourself that you are not a smoker anymore. You have nothing to do with smoking, that you are a new person, and that you are like a snake with a new skin after it has shed its old one.

Whenever I had the urge to smoke, when I was on the edge of going to my neighborhood's mini market to buy cigarettes, I would chew on toothpicks. I would also cut plastic straws into smaller pieces and then chew on them. Also, I would, of course, eat or drink; I would imagine I was on a plane traveling to an exotic destination and I would remind myself that smoking is forbidden on the aircraft.

I would hug myself and go and lay in my bed, singing or thinking about something else until the addictive urge went away. I would close my ears with my hands and scream difficult words until the need to smoke left.

I did all of those things day in and day out until the urge was not as intense as it had been during the first week. I could feel the level of my addiction fading away, which only made me stronger, both mentally and emotionally. After the first two weeks, I realized that it would be even easier and that I would beat this thing; finally, I would be victorious.

My Father's Tactic

While I preferred to chew on toothpicks and drinking straws, my father used another way to fight the urges: he would chew gum. Like me, he would also eat and drink instead of smoking.

Keep a Journal

I made a calendar on May 19th, 2009 to May 19th, 2010; every smoke-free day, I would note it on the calendar. Keeping a diary gave me a sense of duty, and it strengthened my resolve to go through with stopping smoking.

I also started writing a diary. In the beginning, I wrote daily. It helped me a lot to keep going and not give up.

After about six months of being a non-smoker, I stopped writing in it, but it had fulfilled its purpose.

I concluded that if I could last for a year without smoking, then I would be 100% sure that I would stay a non-smoker for life. Now, I made those assumptions based on thinking that if I could manage to be smoke-free through all social situations. Like going out for a coffee with friends who smoke, going to a club where I would have a drink, hanging out after lunch or dinner, or after I had sex—then my brain would make new neuron connections, showing me a life without smoking. I knew I had to retrain myself to live a smoke-free lifestyle.

You need to go through your life as a non-smoker for a year (because one year will cover almost all of the things you used to do when you were a smoker), which will show you that it is possible to get through every situation you encounter in normal life without smoking.

Feeling Invincible

I remember that in the summer of 2009, my best friend and I enjoyed a week in Prague. If you haven't visited Prague, please go or at least put it on your bucket list. The city vista was one of the most beautiful I ever seen in my life, I almost cried. The cleanliness was fantastic, there were so many things to see, and Prague has a lot of towers, which I found surprising. We went in June, which was about 30 to 40 days after I quit smoking. My sinuses had opened, and I could smell again. I felt better because my sleep improved, and I could breathe normally again for the first time after a long time. I also felt more energy without being able to explain why.

There wasn't a single tower or tower clock in Prague where I didn't climb the stairs to the top. Just a few days before visiting

Prague, I had almost collapsed from running up a small hill at my house, but now I was climbing 200 to 300 steps in one breath. It was a pleasant experience, and it helped me see what I had been missing when I had been a miserable smoker.

My friend, who was a smoker at the time, had to use the elevator or when there was none, he would wait at the bottom of the tower for me.

Make A Big Deal Out of It

Then September came, and I celebrated my first smoke-free birthday since I had started. I felt great, to be honest. Every time I saw someone smoke, whether in real life or the movies or TV shows, the craving was there, but it was getting smaller and smaller every day it passed. Although the nicotine was gone from my system, the psychological cravings remained, partly because of my associations with the feel, the smell, and the sight of a cigarette and the ritual of obtaining it, lighting it, and handling it. Those actions and sensations were linked in my mind to the pleasurable effects of smoking, which is what made me crave it.

That's why I was convinced that if I could last a year, then my mind would see that I could live without smoking and know that it was only psychological.

Nicotine, A Deadly Poison

Nicotine is found in the tobacco plant, and it is the natural protection of the plant so it won't get eaten by insects. Its widespread use as an insecticide for crops is now being blamed for killing honey bees. A toxin, drop for drop, nicotine has proven to be as lethal as strychnine and, in studies performed on animals, is now three times deadlier than arsenic.

Some Nasty Info about Nicotine

Nicotine is highly addictive. The ingestion of nicotine results in a discharge of epinephrine from the adrenal cortex, causing a sudden release of glucose. Stimulation is followed by depression and fatigue, leading the abuser to seek more nicotine.

Nicotine is a highly toxic chemical. In rats, a dose of 50 mg per kg is lethal; in mice, the median lethal dose is around 3 mg per kg; and in humans, the median lethal dose is 0.5 to 1.0 mg/kg (or around 40 to 60 mg in an average person).

This little lethal dose makes nicotine more toxic than many other compounds, even including alkaloids such as cocaine, which has a median lethal dose of 95.1 mg per kg in mice.

Nicotine can be absorbed into the bloodstream quickly through the skin. If a highly high concentration of nicotine is spilled on the skin, this can lead to toxicity and death.

What Helped Me Stop Smoking

1.   A healthy state of mind. You should want to quit smoking, and you must not have any doubts about what is your goal and why are you doing it.

2.   Stopping for you. You should not stop as a favor for someone else. If you don't quit smoking for yourself, then you will start smoking again once the conditions that led you to stop return again.

3.   Quit smoking with a friend, a family member, or a group of people. The mutual emotional support is invaluable.

4.   Announcing to everyone you know that you are going to stop smoking: family, friends, colleagues, and others. It's positive peer pressure.

5.   Removing anything that reminds you of smoking (whether in your car or house): lighters, matches, ashtrays, pipes, machines that roll cigarettes, snuff boxes. Get rid of them all, even if some of them were presents from loved ones. Throw all smoking paraphernalia in the trash.

6.   Buy some chewing gum(nicotine free), toothpicks or drinking straws to chew on (or eat and drink instead of smoking; you might gain a few pounds, but your goal is to stop smoking, so you can worry about nutrition and live an otherwise healthy lifestyle later). Try not to replace smoking with food; a few pounds is okay to gain but do not let yourself go and use food as a crutch for quitting smoking.

7.   Making a list of things to do instead if the strong cravings and urges come knocking your door (and then follow through).

8.   Creating a calendar and crossing off every day that you are smoke-free. Write how you felt during craves and what did you do to overcome them. Read each previous entry log before you go to bed.

9.   Keeping a diary to write down how you feel will help you with your confidence (and yes, guys can do this, too; it's not girly to keep a diary).

I hope sharing my smoking and stopping experience helps you to quit smoking or at least think about quitting smoking. Remember, no matter how many years it's been, it's never too late to change. Here is a list of what happens after you stop smoking; the effects are phenomenal:

Within 20 Minutes

Your blood pressure returns to its usual level.

Your pulse rate slows to normal.

Your circulation has improved enough that your hands and feet warm to normal body temperature.

Within 4 Hours

Half of the carbon monoxide from your last cigarette has left your bloodstream.

Within 8 Hours

The carbon monoxide of your last cigarette is now left your blood. Your blood now carries an average amount of oxygen.

Within 24 Hours

Your chance of a heart attack becomes lower.

Within 48 Hours

Damaged nerve endings start to re-grow.

Your sense of smell and taste improve.

Within 2 Weeks to 3 Months

Your circulation becomes better.

Walking and physical activity becomes easier.

Lung function increases up to thirty percent.

Within 1 to 9 Months

You cough less.

You have more energy.

You don't become short of breath as quickly.

The cilia in your lungs re-grow, and you will have less phlegm and infection.

Within 1 Year

Your heart attack risk has fallen to the halfway mark between that of a current smoker and that of someone who has never smoked.

Within 5 Years

If you used to smoke a pack a day, you have now cut your risk of dying of lung cancer in half.

Your risk of heart attack and stroke approaches that of a non-smoker.

You have cut your risk of mouth, throat, and esophageal cancer by half.

Within 10 Years

Your chance of dying from lung cancer is almost as small as a non-smoker's.

Your risk of mouth, throat, esophageal, kidney and pancreatic cancer continues to diminish.

Within 10 to 15 Years

Your risk of dying from any cause is almost the same as that of someone who never smoked.

Lifestyle Changes

After reading a lot about nutrition, especially how to heal yourself by changing your diet, one of the first things I sat down and searched for was what kind of food I should eat and what else I could do to help my lungs and respiratory system, in general, to detoxify faster. I came up with this list:

1. Eat lots of fruits and vegetables. At least 9 servings of fruit and veggies a day.

2. The cleaning nutrients in garlic, onion, ginger, barley grass, kelp, and green tea help with your lungs.

3. Drink lots of water.

4. Drink herbal tea, such as fenugreek, thyme, or cardamom. Green tea is a powerful antioxidant that helps to fight the damage to the lungs.

5. Gradually increase your exercise level; exercise will force your lungs to start working again. Deep breathing and increased blood flow to the lungs will help eliminate and remove some of the toxins.

6. Get enough vitamin A. Check out what your recommended dietary allowance (RDA) is for your age, sex, weight, medical condition, etc.

Sad Mathematics

Before I close this first book of the series about how to quit smoking, I want to go through with you an average evaluation of how many years of my life I lost by smoking.

Let's assume that on an average day, I smoked 40 cigarettes, which is a good estimate of my past smoking addiction.

365 days in a year, times 40 cigarettes per day, equal 14,600 cigarettes a year.

I smoked for 16 years; if we multiply 14,600 cigarettes per year by 16, we get a total of 233,600 cigarettes smoked!

Now we multiply 233,600 cigarettes by 11, which is the number of minutes that you cut your life short with every cigarette you smoke, that gives us 2,569,600 minutes. We divide that by 60 to find out how many hours which is 42826.67 hours. Divide that by 24, and we have 1784.44 days. Divide that by 365, and we have approximately 4.89 years lost from smoking.

I have lost almost five years of my natural life because of smoking, which was an addiction that offered me nothing and was robbing me of my health.

I only hope that with my running habit, which I started back in 2010, I will gradually get back those years with my good health. I also hope that my vegan diet will help to keep me healthy.

How much money did I spend on average on cigarettes during those 16 years of smoking? A pack of cigarettes is, on average, about 4.80 Euros now, so by dividing the number of cigarettes. I smoked (233,600 cigarettes) by the number in each pack (20 cigarettes), we get 11,680 packets; multiply that by 3, and we get 35,040 Euros ($35,040) on average that I spent to kill myself! I sure would love to have that kind of money saved in the bank rather than have smoked it.

Now, these numbers are without calculating the interest if I had that money in the bank!

I am not saying you are going to get wealthy with the money you save from smoking but it sure feels great when the end of the month comes and I have an extra 150 to 250 Euros!

Interesting Calculators

The following list is made up from various calculators that I am sure you will find fascinating.

1.   Free Online Quit Smoking Statistics Calculator (In my book, this is the best calculator I checked out thus far)

http://whyquit.com/free-quit-smoking-meter-calculator.html

2.   How much money you will save calculator.

https://smokefree.gov/how-much-will-you-save

3.   How long will I live is a cool calculator

https://www.myabaris.com/tools/life-expectancy-calculator-how-long-will-i-live/

4.   Smoking Risk Calculator

http://www.medindia.net/patients/calculators/ciger_smoke.asp

5.   Quit Smoking Meter

http://www.calculators.org/health/quit-smoking.php

6.   Cost of Smoking Cigarettes Calculator

https://www.healthstatus.com/calculate/smc

Chapter Epilogue

This first book of the series means a lot to me because smoking was a big part of my life—sixteen years, to be exact. I started smoking when I was 19, and I stopped when I was 35. That's a lot of years! I can't compare it with my father, who was a heavy smoker for 42 years!, but I am very glad that I stopped smoking, because as good luck would have it, my father stopped smoking, too. I am happy that I helped him to get rid of this awful disease and I also respect him for helping me, too.

My intentions here are to inform people, smokers, ex-smokers, and even non-smokers about the nicotine trap and how to escape it for the smokers, how not to fall back in for the ex-smokers, and also how not to get caught by it for the non-smokers. I give this book for free because I want to help people with tobacco smoking, so if you find it interesting, then a good review will help me a lot as a writer.

Chapter 2
Why Do You Smoke?

Prologue

In the first chapter, I told my story as I remember it and of course, it was based on the knowledge I had accumulated and experiences I had until 2014. That's when I started writing my first book Thirsty for health, and a significant portion of the first chapter is derived and based on the chapter Smoking of Thirsty of Health.

Since then two whole years have passed, and in those two years I watched numerous videos by cessation smoking instructors like Joel Spitzer, read numerous articles about tobacco use and nicotine addiction and also read lots of books from people that have the most success with quitting smoking and helping other people quit smoking forever. Also, my experiences analyzed and reran in my head through the new prism of knowledge I acquired gave birth to new conclusions and new information.

I even wrote a book about the rationalizations smokers make to continue smoking, inspired by my experience of smoking for sixteen years and my smoke-free life since 2009.

I entitled it 16 Common Smoking Rationalizations, Recognized, Analyzed and Ultimate Destroyed!

From the tender age of nineteen until the age of thirty-five, the most productive and useful years of a person's life, mine was robbed by a severe deadly drug addiction. I let a drug substance like nicotine hijack the best years of my youth, I open the door and is something I wish I had never done!

In this second book of these series I want to present to you my dear reader something that I wished I knew when I was trying to quit smoking, maybe all of those failed attempts would never have happened if I was informed of the stuff I am aware now.

Everything happens for a reason, and I am a strong advocate of this saying. By learning the way I learn, the order of the life events that happen to me as quitting smoking is concerned prepared me to be able to write this book, so you dear reader will enjoy the benefits of my labor and the lessons from my mistakes! All those failed attempts of quitting smoking did not happen without merit; they were a significant part of my learning experience also.

In this book, I will cover four essential and vital, crucial areas that someone that wants to quit smoking should know. Also if you are not a smoker but want to help a relative or a friend to stop smoking this information are also useful to you too. I am guessing you are a smoker that tried a lot of methods and paraphilia to quit and was not successful. The fact that you are reading my book to me shows only one thing, and that is that you are determined to quit smoking. I hope this book series will give you what you need and want to be able to break free from the nasty and deadly addiction of nicotine.

If you tell someone in general terminology how something is done but without showing to that person in detailed steps how to do it then his or her chances of success are not very high. Or if you indeed show someone how to do something down to the last detail, but you don't explain to him or her why they should do it then again there is a significant chance of failure.

Human beings need two things to achieve anything; they need to understand why are they doing something, what's the purpose, the theory behind it and then show them in practical terms (practice does make perfect) how to do it. You need to give them the why's and show them the how's if you want them to be successful and this is what I am attempting to do with this second book of the series.

So with no further delay, I am presenting to you and also answering the next four paramount life-saving, informative and valuable questions that will enable you to initiate and maintain a smoke-free and nicotine free life, full of health and happiness. The questions are:

1. *Why do you smoke?*

2. *Why should you quit?*

3. *How to stop?*

4. *How to stay off?*

After you read this book, if the information that you acquired resonates with you then your chances of quitting smoking increases dramatically towards a high rate of success. With no further ado let's start the journey that hopefully will enable you to commit to a decision that will lead to a healthy and happy smoke-free life away from sickness, illness, and disease, away from a deadly addiction like nicotine really is.

Why do you smoke?

When I was a miserable smoker from the young age of 19 until the age of 35 non-smokers will always ask me why do I smoke? And my usual response was because I like it! I had other replies, of course, like because I enjoy it, or because it helps me with my stress, or because it helps me wake up in the morning or because it makes my coffee drinking more pleasurable or-or-or.....

All of the above statements are of course subjective, and through the point of view and the mental eye of a smoker it does make sense, and in their head, as it was with me when I was a smoker, they are right.

Of course now more than seven years after my successful quit and being smoke-free I know better. All the above answers I was giving were, of course, false. At the time that I was giving them I thought they were right, but no they were false, truthful on one end of the spectrum but false on the other end of it.

Now the thing I am going to say might not sit well with you, but it's the truth. There is a saying that says: not many people like poetry and truth is like poetry not many people like it at first.

You need to understand that you are a drug addict, I know you don't like the sound of that, but that's the truth, I didn't like it either when I realized it. It doesn't matter that nicotine is legal to buy and distribute and no, Governments all around the world do not care if a product is healthy or not for their populations, they are biased and intertwined with the economic interests of multinational companies like tobacco companies are. So do not make the rationalization that because it is legal, it must be ok to consume, no. Nicotine is a powerfully addictive and deadly substance, and anyone that is using it either through cigs or other delivery methods like vaping, chewing gum or patch is a nicotine addict, in essence, a drug addict.

It's important to understand this concept and start accepting it because it will save your life. The sooner you accept this simple fact the simple truth that you are a drug addict, the faster and easier will be for you to quit smoking by formulating a way to successfully stop smoking thus getting rid of your body the addictive agent namely nicotine.

You smoke because you are a drug addict, and your drug is nicotine.

When you accept that and let it sink into your mindset and allow your conscious self to process it and acknowledge it then you might reach that aha moment, the realization moment will come quicker having as a result of quitting smoking faster and more efficiently. You will reach your aha moment of what are you doing to yourself and wake up from the dream. Not a dream per se but more like a nightmare of what you were doing to yourself all this time with smoking.

Why did I start smoking?

A lot of people including me assumed and still assume that if they figure out why they started smoking that somehow will help them quit smoking faster or easier or both.

The reality of the matter is that the reason you started smoking and the reason you continue smoking have nothing to do with each other.

There are a lot of reasons why someone would start smoking. When I was growing up in Cyprus every man smoke, my father smoked, my grandfather smoked, my uncles, smoked, a lot of my elementary and high school teachers smoked so it was inevitable that at some point I would start smoking too. As a kid watching adults using tobacco the idea in my mind was indoctrinated that when you smoke you are an adult, you are a grown up you are older you are wise you are mature and smart. All these subliminal messages do find their way into kids minds.

The reason I started smoking was pure desperation; something happened when I was doing my military service which at that particular narrow period was lead me to the false impression that my life as I knew it ended. So I said F@ck it and light one, that was it for me I got hooked on nicotine.

Other reasons why someone will start smoking is normal pressure from the immediate environment like your friends, they all smoke, and you feel pressured to start smoking, so you fit in.

Another reason is the rebellious nature of the young; it's expected as reverse psychology debates to do exactly the opposite.

If a teacher tells a child not to start smoking and later in the day the same kid sees his teacher smoke what do you think it will do? If everybody in the adult "gang" tells a youngster not to smoke, and then later all the adults smoke what do you think the youngster will do? You need to lead by example, not just with words.

People started smoking to spite their parents to make other adults of their environment angry, they start smoking out of pure curiosity, started smoking because they thought it's a neat habit. Which is not it's a deadly addiction and the notion smoking is a bad habit is what sends to their grave premature million of people every year on this beautiful planet.

The reason that I continue smoking was not that my life was going to end as I knew it but because in a moment of weakness and stupidity I introduce in my body one of the deadliest addictive drugs on this planet, namely NICOTINE!

I was a drug addict for sixteen years, and I didn't know it, I was under the false impression that I was participating in a ritualistic daily bad habit and not a deadly addiction.

All the reasons I mentioned earlier on how someone started smoking do not have anything to do with the reason you continue smoking. Let me repeat that the reason someone keeps smoking is that that person is a drug addict and needs to satisfy his addiction cravings so he or she will not reach to the point to feel withdrawal symptoms, anything else is hocus pocus and misinformation.

The law of addiction:

The law of dependency as was termed by Joel Spitzer a few decades ago states that if you give to a former addict, the addictive substance he or she was using he or she will become an addict again and return to their previous drug usage.

A lot of you will roll your eyes and question this law not because is not true but what it's doing here a book about smoking. Smoking Is not an addiction many will say it's a bad habit. Unfortunately, it is an addiction and the, unfortunately, is for all those millions of people who have died thus far and are going to die every year because they treat smoking as a bad habit and not as it is a deadly drug addiction.

A small piece of historical fact here about why so many people still think that smoking is a bad habit. This false notion was one of the reasons that my previous attempts failed because I was looking of smoking as a bad habit I had and not as it is, in reality, a deadly addiction.

I searched it further, and I found the answer in one of Joel Spitzer videos. It turns out that On January 11, 1964, Luther L. Terry, M.D., Surgeon General of the United States, released Smoking and Health: Report of the Advisory Committee of the Surgeon General of the Public Health Service. In this famous report, smoking was clearly stated as a habit and not as an addiction, and the reason was that back in 1964 and two years before the launch of Star Trek series. I know I am a Trekkie I tend to use it as a " time landmark" (wink).

More than half of the male population of United States were smokers, and you just couldn't go and announce to the public that smoking is an addiction. If they did say that they would be effectively calling more than half of the male population of United States drug addicts!!!.

Of course, a lot of years later in 1988, the General Surgeon published a new report entitled: *Nicotine Addiction* setting the truth about smoking.

The sad truth is that not many people know either of these reports, the panel of doctors that created the report of 1964 they were all smokers, and many of them including the general surgeon quit after issuing that statement because as doctors knew that it was deadly.

Many people until today are under the impression that smoking is a habit because that's what they hear from other people smokers or nonsmokers. One of the reason is that the tobacco companies whenever there is the issue of smoking and nicotine addiction instead of referencing the 1988 report they conveniently reference the 1964 report where smoking is termed as a habit, and they do that for obvious reasons.

That's how many teenagers get hooked if the kids knew that they are dealing with an addiction that kills one in two and not just an upright habit then they would have a better defense mechanism to say no.

Continuing about the addiction definition, I mean everybody knows that an ex-alcoholic is going to return to his addiction even with the tiniest sip of alcohol. A heroin addict will go back

42

if he injects heroin into its veins. We are very aware of the other drug addictions and how you can be an addict again, but with smoking, there is this apathy, this denial.

Unfortunately for many reasons, we don't see smoking as it is a drug addiction. First is legal and in the minds of many people that means it's ok health wise I mean the government will never allow something that is not okay for you to be sold legally and freely amongst us and worst to our kids and youth. WRONG, governments don't give and excuse my French a flying F@ck about your health all they care about our taxes.

Second, for many years you would see commercials on Tv and also in movies everybody was smoking giving smoking an absolute mystery and sophistication which is not real.

You do not become an adult if you smoke or smarter or more sophisticated you become another statistic a mortal statistic!

Heart attack or stroke, or lung cancer or emphysema and much more "good" things cigarette smoking give you!

That's why when people announce to their friends and family that they quit smoking but see them smoke one or two a few days later do not judge them as harshly as they would judge other addictions like alcohol for example. If you saw a family member or a friend who was an alcoholic having a drink you be in her/his case for doing that because you know it only needs a sip to go back to full-blown alcoholism.

Why don't we have the same attitude towards smoking and we allow relapsing of smoking cigs as something normal? Because we don't see smoking as a drug addiction that's why and I explained why earlier with the general surgeon report.

Next time you see a friend that announced that he quit smoking and catch him or her smoke one or two get on their case. Tell them that this is not right to say that if you quit you quit either you are a smoker (the number of cigs or years of smoking doesn't really matter), or you are not.

Tell them to stop kidding themselves and make a decision, smoker or nonsmoker, an addict or a recovering addict for life. Be strict with them and do not pad them on the back saying its ok you only had one, that one could be the one that will kill him or her at the end. That one will take him or her back to full-blown smoking and down the road in one, five, ten or fifteen years it will kill them!

Quitting smoking is not something to take light or joke about it's an effort to stop a drug addiction a deadly drug addiction, and it should get the seriousness it deserves both from the person who is doing the quitting and also the people that support him or her.

You need to understand that quitting smoking is a process that its ultimate goal is to break free from a DRUG addiction and not a meaningless not so important habit. It's a FIGHT for your life, and you should be committed 100% to it.

Why should you quit?

I should start answering this question with the following sentence. Unfortunately, the first sign of some of the smoking-related illnesses is sudden death!

More Americans are dying from tobacco every year than all the Americans killed in world war II!

Every 18 months more Americans die than all the wars of the 20th century combined (World War I. World War II, Korea and Vietnam, Gulf War)

50% of smokers die prematurely, and the rest 50% end up having a crippling condition like emphysema. The ages of the smokers that die are also shocking from 35 to 69 years old; that's like 20 to 40 years of life expectancy lost. Tobacco kills around 6 million people each year. More than 5 million of those deaths are the result of direct tobacco use while more than 600 000 are the result of non-smokers being exposed to second-hand smoke. Nearly 80% of the world's 1 billion smokers live in low- and middle-income countries.

The primary reason smokers prematurely die is not cancer but from heart diseases. Cancer and the most recognized cancer lung cancer are the second reason. There are many more diseases that are caused by smoking except the lungs, other places of the human body where cigarettes inflict carcinogenic effects are lips, tongue, mouth, larynx, esophagus, and pharynx. In addition to the previously mentioned cancers, cigarettes are blamed for diseases of the bladder, pancreas, kidney, and stomach.

The third reason smokers die again prematurely cutting their life expectancy sometimes in half is stroke and the mechanism that causes a stroke is the same as the one that causes fatal heart diseases. The fourth reason is accidents, some accidents that most people do not associate with smoking like car accidents and fire.

When I was a smoker the only bit of information, I knew about smoking was that I might get lung cancer. I was oblivious to the fact that more people die from cardiovascular diseases attributed to smoking than lung cancer.

I don't know why a lot of individuals associate smoking more with cancer, while most of the smokers die from cardiocirculatory situations caused by cigarette smoking than from diseases inflicted by cigarettes.

I was surprised when I found out that nicotine is the primary culprit of heart diseases and strokes. Even after more than seven years without smoking I still thought that the only danger from smoking was various cancers. It's my research I made and still making about the book I wrote 16 Common Smoking Rationalizations, Recognized, Analyzed and Ultimate Destroyed! That opened my eyes to the real dimensions of tobacco use and its deadly grip that has on smokers around the globe.

The webpage of the W.H.O. organization says it in black and white that effects on our cardio-circulatory system are both fast-induced, immediate and severe.

Nicotine is the evil here, except being the addictive substance, the one that holds our freedom away is also a potent stimulant responsible for raising our heart rate, blood pressure and also responsible for the constriction of our arteries. Wow was the first word that came out of my mouth when I learned that. This means that all those people that are using NRT's (Nicotine Replacement Therapies) are still in great danger of losing their life prematurely from cardiovascular illnesses and circulatory problems including heart attack and stroke.

The other significant major contributor to cardiovascular diseases and also stroke is carbon monoxide which with the help of nicotine, cause a condition to your body called atherosclerotic. Atherosclerosis is a Greek word, and it means the deposit of a pulp like substance inside the arteries reducing the blood flow. In other words, it means hardening of the arteries.

What is Atherosclerosis?

Atherosclerosis in more medical terms is an illness where the plaque is accumulated internally in your arteries. Now for those who don't know what arteries are, arteries are blood vessels of various sizes which have a very significant task which is to carry blood rich in oxygen to our heart and other parts of our body. If you search for "human circular system" in any search engine machine, you will get a photo of the human body with thousands of arteries running through it, and that will give you an idea of the grandeur of the human body and of the importance of the circular system.

Now plaque is made off from fat, cholesterol, calcium, and other elements that are found in the blood. With time, the plaque narrows and hardens the smoker's arteries. This has as a direct result the limit of the flow of the blood that is carrying the oxygen to our organs and other members of the smoker's body.

Atherosclerosis can cause some dangerous situations, which are a stroke, heart attack, and even death!

I am giving you a list of atherosclerosis-Related Diseases

Coronary Heart Disease

Carotid Artery Disease

Peripheral Artery Disease

Chronic Kidney Disease

The clogging process of atherosclerosis creates problems to the heart and to other parts of the smoker's body like the brain and peripheral blood circulation in the extremities of the smoker's body. Sometimes this constriction of the arteries results to gangrene and amputations of the extremities of the smoker! They lose feet and hands! (Buerger's Disease)

If you are still not convinced that you need to quit smoking, then here are some more reasons of why you should quit smoking. Most people who are ready to accept the truth already searched and knew a lot of what I just mentioned, but this is me just being thorough about it so here are some more reasons People Want to Quit Smoking are:

1.   Complication of preexisting conditions

2.   Complications in post-operative and anesthesia situations.

3.   Individuals and generally society is more informed about what smoking is, so there is more pressure on smokers than before, that's why there is a phenomenon in these days of the so-called closet smoker.

4.   The act of smoking is offensive and disgusting is you analyze it. It is smelly, teeth and hands become yellow, clothes reek with smoke the skin gets wrinkled and ages faster.

5.   A woman in the old days would see a beautiful woman in black, white movies smoke, and they thought wow I could be beautiful too if I start smoking, or men will see macho men smoke and pick up smoking thinking they would be like them, sharp and sophisticated. Well, society now does not believe smoking is modern anymore on the contrary society believes that smokers are people that cannot control themselves and are looked down upon and many times scorned for their smoking.

6.   Think of all the money you are wasting away, think of all the things you can do with that extra money in your pocket. Many said including myself that if the pack goes 3 Euros, I quit, well the package went to be 4.5 Euros, and I was still smoking because I was a drug addict, addicts don't think like that. Today an average price for a pack of cigs in Cyprus anyway is about 4 Euros. Multiply that by 365 days is 1560 Euros a year! Just think of that? And if both smoke husband and wife that's 3120 Euros a year going down the drain.

7.   Smokers start fires, but they also make holes to their clothes some of those clothes are expensive.

Now continuing my arguments of why you should quit, When I was a smoker, I was always smoking in the car and the times that I manage to throw hot ash on my lap were numerous.

I can't remember how many times I was trying to remove the ash from my lap or my seat and not paying attention to the road!

The numbers I could have had an accident, either killing other people or destroying my car and injuring myself. Even worse lose my life because instead of driving carefully I was behaving like a typical drug addict.

The other thing smokers do while they drive, I personally never done that, is to throw their cigarette out of the window because they don't want to make a mess of the cars ashtray and they must clean it. Sometimes when they do that the wind brings the cig's bud back into the car from the open window of the back seat and minutes later, they are distracted because the back seat is on fire! Another thing that could happen is to start a forest fire destroying the natural environment and many times destroying the homes of people that live near, around or into the woods!

I always used the ashtray of the car to extinguish the cig; I always did that because I had a sense of forest fires starting like that, so I was more conscious about it. Of course, the car stung like a chimney, but I was oblivious to it, my smell sense was not operational. Next time you are in a traffic jam and smokers start smoking notice what they do when they finish the cig they will most probably throw it out the window without thinking.

Stress Symptoms

The reason a smoker smokes while in a traffic jam is that their stress level goes up because he is in a hurry to go somewhere to do something. He is stressed out that he will not get on time and will not achieve his work and that creates an accumulative effect on its stress and anxiety level.

As I mentioned on numerous other occasions here stress makes your urine more acidic, and the body takes the nicotine in the smoker's bloodstream and flashes it down into the urine to make them more alkaline. This has a result of the extensive removal of nicotine from the body making the smoker to have severe withdrawal symptoms thus lighting a cig to reestablish the desired nicotine levels into the blood, so the withdrawal symptoms will stop.

Notice that when a smoker is really stressed if she has the chance she will light a cig if they don't have a chance you will see that she will be in a state of alertness. Which are the symptoms of early withdrawal from not replenishing the nicotine needed to bring it to the levels that the body through tolerance allows it to be floating in the blood?

Another reason smokers have car accidents is that of the numbness smoking inflicts on them, their response time and reflects slowed down by at least 50% compared to an average person.

Sometimes it's not even the smokers fault, but because of the slow-paced reflexes caused by smoking, they end up killing someone else, destroying his car or even worse end up dead themselves.

Another accident also associated with tobacco use and it's closer to mind to relate fires. I remember that many times I fell asleep in my bed watching TV having a cig in my hands and many times I will wake up because the cig burned my hand and made me awake.

Ashtrays full of extinguished cigs, or that's what I thought, thrown in the trash bin will rekindle and burn the trash bin resulting in a full-blown apartment or house fire. I was lucky that I didn't burn myself alive all those addictive years.

The fourth reason smokers die from is Chronic Obstruction of Pulmonary Diseases in short COPD, which includes emphysema and bronchitis. Two crippling conditions that make the quality of your life a living hell and reduce your ability to breathe normally obstructing you from participating in any athletic activities (playing hide and seek with your kids, making love to your spouse, etc.)

Smoking is the leading cause of emphysema, and there are very rare situations where someone could have emphysema without smoking because she may lack a particular enzyme but that's rare. The vast bulk of emphysema is smoking tobacco related. Emphysema is not the lack of ability to inhale which that's what most people think, on the contrary, it's the inability of the person to exhale. The reason is that years of smoking has a result, the destruction of the lungs shape and also the crippling of the lungs elasticity.

Imagine a balloon being filled with air then if you want to remove the air, you let the nozzle free, and the balloon shrinks back to its size removing the air out. That's what the lung can't-do anymore or does it with great difficulty; the lungs cannot return to their normal shape because first, they lost their elasticity and second their shape is ruined by the 4000 chemicals that make up the TAR of a cigarette!

You can imagine how a person with emphysema feels like with the following example. Take a deep breath and hold it and without exhaling try to breathe some more, hold that too, without exhaling try to breathe again for the third time.

How and what you felt while trying to breathe the second and third time that's how a person with emphysema feels every time she wants to do something natural like breathing. Tobacco smoking takes his breath away literally!

Imagine living for ten, twenty even thirty years with emphysema! It just doesn't worth it.

The sixth leading cause smokers die off is Pneumonia and Influenza. The lungs have a defensive mechanism called cilia which in very lame terms are thousand little brooms of the lungs. If you have a viral or a bacterial infection the body with the help of cilia removes the mucus eliminating the bacteria and virus out of the system and keeps our lungs and our body in strong shape and optimized condition.

Smoking paralyzes and destroys the cilia resulting in the body inability to remove excess mucus filled with poisons, toxins, and bacteria with the consequence being to get flu and diseases more often. The immune system's ability to remove the mucus because of the destruction of cilia makes the smokers more prone to illness and diseases.

While I was smoking, I had chest pains, and I was coughing a lot especially in the morning right after waking up. I remember I would spit green and yellow substances. Being asleep for some hours and mainly not smoking gave my body some time to do its work which was to get rid of the toxins I was poisoning it daily. Toxins like nicotine and another 4000 chemicals that constitute tar.

The first thing I was doing when I was waking up to put a cig in my mouth poisoning and killing myself even more, but then again a drug addict doesn't care about that? He only cares to get its fix, to get the addictive agent that will keep him away from any possible "dreaded" withdrawal symptoms.

That was my symptoms, and it should have told me that hey stupid wake up you are killing yourself with this cig smoking just stop it.

But no, human nature, we think that nobody and nothing will hurt us, that others will get that cancer or emphysema, not us we are invincible.

There are so many signs that our body is trying to tell us that smoking is not good for us. Smokers a cough on a daily basis, have shortness of breath, hoarseness you know someone is s smoker by his damaged vocal cords, chest pains, cold or tingling in extremities, and digestive disorders. I am positive that smoking was a massive contributor to my stomach and duodenum ulcer except for inadequate nutrition of course and finally fatigue.

All these warning signals do not make or convince the smoker to stop because as I said they are waiting for something to happen to quit or using false rationalizations to convince themselves that smoking has nothing to do with their cold or flu or bronchitis, so they will continue smoking.

Well I was one of the lucky ones, and you can be too if you wish, I quit before something happened to me. I didn't have to stop because something happened to me. One thing that could happen is sudden death, and then you SURE quit smoking for GOOD!

Sudden death is a big possibility with smoking just keep that in mind the next time you put a cig in your mouth thinking I am still healthy I can keep smoking. Also, sudden death while smoking can occur without any warning signs, one moment you are there, father, a mother, a husband a wife and the next a dead, lifeless, cold corpse that people put in a coffin and downloading it into a grave! Did I draw a graphic picture for you yet?

The method of harm reduction

Government medical agencies and the medical establishment promotes the false idea that quitting smoking is really hard. When I was 24 years old, I was already smoking for 5 years, and this notion that quitting smoking was hard was engraved in my mind. Also, everybody was telling me exactly that. Quitting smoking is hard, it's hard it's not easy you will need help to stop. I had this image of that it takes a lot of effort and too much time to quit.

There is a reason that society thinks like this and it's because it's being influenced and bombarded by commercials of NRT's that they promise to alleviate the pain of quitting smoking or make your quit easier by making the so-called harm reduction.

54

Quitting smoking cigs and replacing it with an NRT or even an e-cig might reduce the danger of a lung cancer because 4000 chemicals that are in the smoke are not getting into your lungs anymore. But, nicotine is not innocent as the vast majority of people think, it's responsible for more than 50% of the deaths annually on this planet that's roughly 2,5 million inhabitants!

Nicotine is an artery restriction agent, meaning it blocks and clogs your arteries giving you heart attacks and strokes!

Why will you put yourself in a so-called harm reduction plan and not remove the harm entire from your life by going cold turkey in the first place?

How to stop?

My adamant opinion is that going cold turkey is the only way to quit smoking. Yes, of course, there are other ways and methods, but the vast majority of people that quit tobacco use and were successful made it with the Cold Turkey method. The Cold Turkey method says just stop smoking and not using any NRT's or cutting gradually down. COLD TURKEY is the most successful method, it was the manner that allowed me to quit successfully back in 2009 and I am still smoke-free. Also it was the way I used instinctively in my previous attempts except for the first one which was with nicotine patches.

If you listen to your body, the only way to get rid of an addiction is to stop delivering to your system the addictive agent, in my case back in 2009 and at your current status dear reader Nicotine. Nicotine addiction is the reason people smoke; it's one of the most powerful chemical substances and a heavy drug in my book. Smoking kills annually more people than all the people that die from the illegal drugs combined!

Now let's see why Cold Turkey method is ideal for you.

Let's see the advantages of cold turkey method:

1. Vast majority used and continued to use this method to quit smoking because it's the natural process your body asks you.

2. It's the cheapest way to stop smoking you don't spend any money on NRT's or other prescribed drugs.

3. It's the safest way to quit smoking, no possible side effects of prescription drugs that supposedly help you quit smoking.

Many you will say to me that I am wrong that there are many ways to quit smoking-yes I will give you that there are many ways but the only way that has the statistics on its side its cold turkey method. All the other methods which I pretty much tried like cutting down, gradually smoking fewer cigs, or NRT's like nicotine patch. Other methods which I did not try like prescription drugs, hypnosis, acupuncture and so many others statistically are not successful methods because their success rate is negligible at best.

I mean do you want to get rid of the addiction once and for all, do you want to be successful do you want to take back your life do you want to be a winner from now on then don't think twice go cold turkey!

How did the person you know quit smoking?

If you don't believe that Cold Turkey is the way to go then my advice is to ask people that are smoke-free for at least a year. Ask them which method and how they quit and you will see after your little poll that Cold Turkey is the winner.

In my first book, Thirsty for Health, I wrote that I asked around how to quit smoking, and a lot of people said use nicotine patches. It was very popular back then and me going with the social notion of stopping I went and bought a nicotine patch package, and I used it for 3 or 4 days. After the fourth day, if I am not mistaken, I started smoking again.

Back then I didn't know anything about smoking, and with the knowledge, I have now it's obvious that I made a few terrible mistakes.

First I believed the words of people telling me that nicotine patch is an effective way of quitting smoking, trust me it is not. Second I didn't ask them if they quit smoking using this method, and third and most important of all I thought quitting smoking was really hard to do and in my head, it was flirting with impossible. You can see that all the odds were against me! I was a walking disaster.

After years when I did a bigger research, and I was a bit more detailed with my investigation, I concluded that the best way to quit smoking was cold turkey, just stop smoking it was that simple. It is the natural way the body asks you to do it, to give your body the chance to do its job which is to clean it from nicotine, allow for the cilia (the natural brooms of our lungs) to start regenerating and working again.

NRT's Nicotine Replacement so-called Treatments do not help you quit smoking; they do not help you escape the nicotine prison they just change the way you continue to be a hooked junkie a drug addict. They change It from a cig to a patch or gum or a spray and so on. Instead of giving away your hard earned money to the tobacco companies you are giving them away to pharmaceutical companies, and you are stuck in the middle again, still inserting toxins in your body still killing yourself slowly and sometimes not that slowly from the inside out.

Also, there was this notion that going cold turkey is the worst way to quit smoking, that's one of the biggest myths ever. It's the worst scenario for the pharmaceutical companies that want you to get hooked on their products; they don't care for your health all they care is their unyielding profits.

More than fifty percent of the planet's smokers are now ex-smokers that tell me that quitting smoking is not that hard, from the moment you have more ex-smokers than smokers that mean is doable and not impossible. That's one thing I learned the second is that it's the method with the most success rate so why again would I choose an NRT method? When the statistics say it in black and white that cold turkey is the best and more successful quitting process and all the people I know including me used that method to clean themselves from the nicotine jail!

I will close this section of my book by repeating and by saying it's the most efficient way to quit smoking, it's cheap doesn't have to buy anything else like the NRT's are asking of you. It's the method used by all the rest of the addictions, like alcohol, cocaine, and heroin.

It's a way that people employed and applied on the spark of the moment they woke up one day, and they realized what they were doing to themselves, others quit smoking because their doctor told them that if they don't, they will die. Others quit smoking because they got the flu or the really bad case of the cold, and they haven't smoked for days, and after they had got well they said hey I haven't smoked in days lets see where this will go and they end up quitting for good!

I remember that every time I would get the flu I wouldn't smoke for at least a week! And I was always wondering how come I can live without smoking? These flu situations along with other realizations helped me get to my aha moment that smoking was not good for me.

How to stay off?

I presented thus far what smoking is which is a drug addiction. I hope, you started the procedure of convincing yourself that you are a drug addict and that your drug is nicotine, this will help you deal any future quitting attempts with better odds of success. I also present why you should quit, the compelling volume of scientific evidence and facts that smoking is a killer is undeniable. If you wish to continue to live in denial, then that's another story, but I am sure if you are a sensible and logical human being you simply cannot ignore them. Finally, I showed you how to quit smoking, and that's by using the Cold Turkey method, the method I use to stop smoking and so many million people around the world. Now the question and one of the most important of the four is how to stay away from smoking.

From experience and all the books and the articles and all the Information I searched and researched how to stay off is more psychological than physiological.

The first days as I will analyze and present in the following books of the series are more related with physiological urges and after the first week without smoking psychological urges are more in play.

How to stay off smoking comes down to a key action which is to never take another puff in your life, like an alcoholic to remain free alcohol addiction mustn't drink even a small sip of alcohol. That's how you stay off smoking, do not buy them, do not accept any cigs from friends family or strangers, just don't put them in your mouth again. Also, do not confuse cigars as something else they are the same they deliver nicotine to your blood as well. Stay away from nicotine gum, patches, sprays, vaping, hookahs electronic cigs, chewing tobacco, etc.

I repeat If you want to stay away from smoking never take another puff ever again.

Smoking is not an option is not a good mantra because smoking is an option and if you want to take that opportunity then for me there are only two reasons why would anyone would want to start smoking again or wants to start smoking.

You want to start smoking until it kills you because that's what smoking does, it might not kill you fast like a fatal heart attack or a fatal stroke, you might end up having lung cancer where you will probably have another 3 to 5 years of life to you before you die. You can get emphysema, and you will not be able to breathe normally for the rest of your life, and you be not able to do anything!

Or you can get pancreatic cancer where in this case in three months you are a goner.

So yes picking up smoking or starting smoking again is a good option for someone that wants to have a life full of diseases, ill health and wants to die sooner than the years he could have on this planet by leading a healthy lifestyle.

The other option an ex-smoker has and would start smoking again is if he or she really enjoyed the withdrawal symptoms then sure you should smoke a cig every three days. Smoking every three days you can have those "excellent" withdrawal symptoms, and that's an amazing way to feel them and have them forever.

Other than that I don't think there are any "good" options to smoke. Your call, your decision, your choice you are an adult, my dear reader.

Just say no to lighting a cigarette but don't stay on the no word, do not make yourself feel that you are saying no to something good or something that offers you or benefits you in any way. Do not deprive yourself because you said no, instead give focus on why you said no, give emphasis on the whole picture, that you are getting away from a deadly addiction and the way to do this at least for the first three days is to say no to lighting a cig. You will see as the time passes the physiological urge will fade away, you will reach a point of epiphany, and you will realize that you are smoke-free. The only way to keep this wonderful feeling is never to take another puff in your life because if you do, then you are away from a pack a day if you are lucky maybe you will smoke more than a pack a day!

A puff a day from a pack a day.

This is a good mantra; it has a logical validity it shows what will happen if you take a puff. You have a significant percentage of starting smoking again.

You need to reinforce your mind with good thoughts positive thoughts, why you are stopping, for your health, for you, for all the money you save.

That's why it's a good tactic to make a list why you are quitting smoking and read them every time you have an urge for smoking.

Just think of something else is a useless advice. When you want a cig, you need to refocus your thoughts on two things first acknowledge the fact that you want a cig does not deny it. Then focus on the reasons that you are quitting smoking, your health, better smell and taste, your breath doesn't stink anymore. Teeth are not going to be yellow anymore, the skin will get healthier and brighter, also if you are a guy and have a goatee or mustache no yellow goatee and mustache anymore!

You will be able to enjoy your food and your coffee better now because your senses are starting to work again and for the first time in years you be able to taste and smell how food tastes and how coffee smells and tastes!

Your clothes will not be saturated and stink of smoke; you be able to start participating in events that are a bit more athletic in nature because your lungs will start using more oxygen, oxygen that was denied because of the carbon monoxide you were inhaling through cigs.

Your heart attack and stroke danger are going to drop because you stop putting nicotine into your bloodstream.

Think of all the money you will be saving and not wasting on smoking.

The bottom line is smarter than nicotine not stronger, every time you have an urge for smoking, recognize it accept it, don't deny it but at the same time reinforce your commitment and resolve to quit by analyzing and reading the reasons you are quitting smoking. Remind yourself why you are stopping tobacco use, and you be ok, trust me I know I being there back in 2009 when I quit smoking. It gets easier with every day you are smoke-free.

Lost long-term quits a beautification term for failure

There are no such things, long-term quits. The notion and the trap that many people start smoking again are because, with time they forget why they quit, they forgot that smoking is addictive, and also they think that they can control it. People that stop tobacco use and are smoke-free for a year need to remind themselves that they are drug addicts in recovery forever and it only needs a small puff to get them back to smoking because the nicotine receptors inside our brain will always be there ready to be satisfied with deadly nicotine.

Remind yourself that you are a recovering drug addict in the morning. Make it the first thing you wake up. Congratulate yourself for not smoking even one cig at the end of every day. That's what I often do, I may not do it every day because I don't think of smoking at all now but I do remind myself that I was a smoker. I remind to myself that it only takes one puff to go back because that's how I became a smoker in the first place I took a puff back in 1993! And it took me sixteen years to come to my senses.

I will quit smoking someday!

From the many failed attempts I had, the attempts that I programmed but never even started and finally from my successful 2009 quit which is still valid I learned that if you don't realize what you are doing to yourself with smoking and also educate yourself on what is nicotine addiction the chances of quitting are minuscule.

They were a time that I was at the beginning of a quit, and I was so sure I would never smoke again; I was so sure that I was willing to bet money but alas I smoke again.

One of the reasons I was failing with my previous quit attempts was that I thought that quitting smoking was just a rational decision on its own, that it's a mental situation I falsely believed that I had a bad habit!

If I knew that I was dealing with an addiction, then I would be better prepared I would know about the physiological withdrawal of nicotine, and I would be more ready psychologically thus increasing my possibilities of a successful quit.

In my mind back then thoughts like it's only a small nasty habit I will get rid of it in no time, but when the physical withdrawal came, I didn't know how to face resulting in ending returning back to smoking.

When you decide to quit smoking you must make a commitment never to put another cig in your mouth and yes psychological, and emotional aspects are important, but we need to be ready for the possible withdrawal effects, so we are better prepared for them.

People will say that is in control of their quit and others will say they are too weak to stop smoking. Most of the times and I know this from experience witnessing friends and other people at work stopping, and I realized that people that have complete control of their lives assume that they can control quitting cigarette with the same fashion. What they lack is understanding that cigarette smoking is a drug addiction and it controls them, Nicotine in a substance level wins every time, it's powerful, and that's why you kept smoking in the first place after that first cig.

What you can do is to recognize that and understand that you need to be smarter than this dangerous product and not stronger, nicotine's IQ is zero nonexistent! Be smarter, not stronger.

People that were complaining that they are weak and that they can never quit are usually the people that manage to quit smoking. Because with every day they go by without a cigarette, their resolve is getting bigger, and they start to see with their own eyes and feel with all their other senses that they can actually pull this off.

I had to go through both of this mindsets in the course of failed attempts, but it helped me realize and understand better what it needs to be done to have a successful quit and finally to stay off smoking forever.

Which day to Quit.

The best day to quit is on a Tuesday, your first day of your quit should be on a Tuesday. Let me explain why. It's a workday, and you must go to work, but the good thing about Tuesday is that it doesn't have the bad vibes of a Monday because it interrupted your weekend.

You will go through your normal routine at work without lighting a cigarette because you already got rid of them the previous day and everything that has any relation to smoking and nicotine addiction.

After work, you will again do everything you were doing the previous Tuesday but now without smoking. You will not think about the future at all, you will be focused and committed to going without a cigarette for this Tuesday only, nothing else should pop into your head, you will face any urges, and possible withdrawal needs as they come.

You will wake up Tuesday morning, and you will not light a cig, you will stand in front of a mirror, and you will say to yourself: This is my first day of freedom from Nicotine!

Sources

http://www.who.int/tobacco/research/heart_disease/en/
https://www.nhlbi.nih.gov/health/health-
topics/topics/atherosclerosis

Chapter 3
First Day Of Your Freedom

First Day – D-day.

If you are reading these lines, it means one thing and one thing only. It means that you took the decision to quit smoking, it means that something inside you made you realize that smoking is offering you nothing, literally nothing.

It kills you from the inside out; the nicotine is messing up your arteries by constricting them and filling them with fat which gradually turns into plague making you a candidate for fatal heart attack and stroke!

The tar of the smoke blackens your lungs and destroys the immune system of your lungs making you more vulnerable to diseases and illness. Furthermore, about 60 to 80 out of the 4000 chemicals that are in the tar are carcinogenic in nature meaning they can cause you cancer.

You are reading these lines because unconsciously you realized all of the above and already made a commitment to stop this addiction, you made the decision and committed yourself to break free from smoking and from the nicotine prison that holds your soul.

The previous two books of the series, have one single goal in mind to give you the weapons and ammunition and the knowledge to help you fight your addiction make your commitment stronger and unyielding, knowledge is power as long it is used wisely and productively.

I am giving you this information that is sprouted from my personal experience of being a pathetic smoker for 16 years and also from quitting smoking and being an ex-smoker since 2009. Having this two different characteristics, I am in a unique position to walk you through from all the phases of the procedures, and I am hopeful you be victorious at the end.

Quitting smoking is easy even if you think right now it is not. The truth is that quitting smoking is super easy to do, keep away from smoking is where your commitment will be tested but following certain philosophies and specific psychological guides you be on your smoke-free life in no time.

I am selling you nothing except my books which do not cost much. If you think you pay 5 dollars and more on average every day to buy your cigs, then my books which will help you quit smoking and get your health and your life back costs nothing in comparison.

Let's begin the catharsis, my dear reader, and I am here to tell you that you just made the first step to a healthier and happier version of you. A journey begins with a small step, I know I was where you are now back in the year 2009. I am sure if you stick with your commitment you will reach the same level of mental clarity and resolution which I enjoy now.

An immediate issue I want you to understand and also will help you dispense the unfounded fears you have when quitting smoking is that the way you will feel or feel right now on day one or the few couple of days after is not going to last forever. It's only temporary until all nicotine will be removed from your body.

One of the first things you should do on your first day of quitting is to throw away anything and everything that has anything and everything with the act of smoking. Namely cigarettes, lighters, matches, pipes if you smoked them, Nicotine Replacement Items like nicotine gum and nicotine patches, sprays, fresh tobacco. Ashtrays get rid of them, start cleaning your life with all these elements of death and do it having in the back of your mind that it is a good thing that you are quitting smoking. It is something that will save your life; you are leaving nothing back literally nothing back except a possible death and crippling life!

Personally back in 2009 when I had my successful quit which still stands I was a bit overzealous when I got rid of all of the smoking-related items. I got rid of all the matches and lighters of the house, and my mother was furious because she could not find a match or a lighter to use to light her gas stove with (oops)

If you have a member of the family that needs matches or lighters asked them politely to keep them away from you and not to leaves them in a public and accessible part of the house. Ask them to do this before the day you decided to quit which is better to be on a Tuesday as I mentioned in the previous book of the series.

Do not make the mistake which I did when I first tried to quit smoking. I locked myself in my apartment for three days being 100% confident that I will not smoke ever again because I would not have any distractions.

It worked for three days I did not smoke, but on the fourth day when I got out of the door to see some of my friends I smoked again, and do you know why? The reason was that I imprisoned myself in four walls without allowing myself to experience and challenge myself to be smoke-free in a real social environment and situation.

When you decide to quit smoking do not lock up yourself in four walls, live your life as you did before. This is the only way to stop smoking because you will have to train yourself to do exactly all the things you did as a smoker but now train and reprogram yourself to do it without using a cigarette.

This is your first day breaking free from smoking, and you should repeat to yourself that it is worth it, today is the day that you are taking your health back and also your life back. Now how severe the withdrawal symptoms will be for you? The truth is nobody knows, and that is the real simple truth, and I want you to know I will always tell you the truth no matter how hard or hurtful or unbelievable you may think it is. Each withdrawal process is different for each person, and also each previous withdrawal symptoms of previously failed quit attempts made by the same individual are also different!

You might have terrible withdrawal symptoms, and you might not even think about smoking while you are on your quit effort, most of the cases the withdrawal symptoms are in between, not too hard not too easy, bearable.

From my experience the more you know about the process of cleaning your body from nicotine the more in control you be, and mental agony and withdrawal symptoms appear to be less in intensity because you are using your *intelligence to beat the addiction*, not your willpower. The important thing to remember is that you need to make a personal commitment never to put another cigarette in your mouth.

If you put one, then it only needs a puff to go back to full grown nicotine addiction. Do not put another cigarette in your mouth ever again.

Also even if you have a very terrible discomfort you have pains and headaches, and you are shaking uncontrollably. I assure you these trouble conditions you are now they will only last for a few days. It's much much more preferable to endure this kind of suffering for a few days instead of the suffering you might endure from the dangers smoking can give you, heart attacks,

71

strokes that might be fatal and also lung cancer and emphysema that will cripple you physically and steal your life away from you. I promise you the pain you might feel now it is only temporary and will not be present for the rest of your life, and it is much better than ending up dying or having your life crippled by smoking. I repeat that so you understand that you might have severe withdrawal symptoms or no symptoms at all! Nobody really knows you will have to find out for yourself.

You are fighting for your life now, *do not take quitting smoking lightly*. It is your LIFE we are talking about now, make the commitment ensure the withdrawal process, remember, it's not going to last forever, with every day without smoking the symptoms will be lighter, and they will disappear eventually I promise you that, back in 2009 I was there where you are now.

You need to be patient and push through, watch the videos and the reading material I suggest and understand that *you are fighting for your life*, you are fighting to win back your health and happiness.

Read the list of actions I advise you to do and also the list of items that you should avoid for the first few days. When I am telling you to avoid certain things to do it is because I know from my experience the urge to smoke will be present, and I am aware that avoiding them in this early phase of detoxification is the smart thing to do, you need to be smarter than nicotine not stronger.

Do not change anything in your day because you are quitting smoking, the sooner you go through your life without smoking the quicker you will see and realize that you can live without tobacco use, stress anxiety and fear of not making the quit will start to disappear gradually, and that is a good thing.

72

My advice as nutrition is a concern and is something I haven't done when I quit smoking because I was ignorant is drink lots of juices the first three days of the effort. If you want to continue after the three days then, by all means, please do, but at least the first three days of the quit drink many natural made juices.

The juice consumption will help you with two things, it will stabilize your blood sugar and will not give you the cravings I had and also it will expedite the removal of nicotine from your body by acidifying the urine thus making nicotine leaving your body faster.

You can control any withdrawal effects with deep breathing, relaxation exercise, and yoga; it is an unusual and very efficient way to deal with the possible withdrawal symptoms.

Your first day is a day you will remember forever it is the day that you took your life back. You should bear in mind that it does not matter how bad It might be but how much important it is for you.

Anybody can quit smoking; I am the living proof of it, you need to believe in yourself. Do not hear what other people say about quitting smoking, everybody can do it, there is no selective few that can pull it off, the number worldwide proves it and what they say is that there are more ex-smokers than smokers on this planet. Now that tells me one thing that smoking is doable and also it does not matter how many failed efforts you had in the past or how many years you smoked or how many cigs you did every day or what everybody else thinks, quitting smoking is very doable, and you can do it! It is possible!

You will notice in my first book of the series I am saying that I belonged to that exclusive 7% of the people that managed to break free from smoking, that was my mindset back in 2014 when I started writing my first book Thirsty for Health. I was basically depicting my past state of mind. I was also reproducing what society thinks about quitting smoking, which is false and deadly erroneous. It is when I started searching and researching for these book series that I found out that this 7 % does not apply, it is something tobacco companies, and pharmaceutical companies and even health organization of various countries argue that makes people think that quitting smoking is hard. They want you to believe that, so you can either continue smoking convinced that it is fatal to quit because it is impossible. The other trap is trying to stop smoking with the so-called NRT's (Nicotine Replacement Therapies) where first will not halt the nicotine addiction since the addictive substance is still circulating in your blood, and instead of giving your hard earned money to the tobacco companies you will start giving them to the pharmaceutical companies.

I am not a conspiracy theorist, but when power and money are involved, you should always keep in mind that public's well-being is never considered, companies make more money on the suffering of people than on the health or happiness of individuals.

Quitting smoking is very easy, and it is easier using the Cold Turkey method, and you can take that to the bank.

How to face the fear of quitting smoking

I had a lot of failed attempts to quit smoking, some of them I mentioned in my first book Thirsty for Health. Every time I was making an effort to stop I had two main fears, the first one and the most obvious was that I would fail again! It was the first thought in my mind, and it was present throughout the procedure. The reason I was failing, of course, was not because of just the fear; I now know that it was because I did not know exactly of what I was dealing with, which is the fact that I was a drug addict. I did not know that or I knew it, but I was in deep denial either way. When you do not know what are you facing, then you do not know how to prepare and deal with it efficiently.

One good thing that came out of the many failed attempts of mine was that with every failed attempt I was learning something new, and I was incorporating it in my next attempt most of the time subconsciously. I was lucky that I was a stubborn man. I am very scholastic, and I tend to search and experiment until I get something perfect. I will do it until I achieve the relevant perfection.

The last piece of knowledge that I acquired and helped me a lot to quit was an article I read on the internet in 2009 that nicotine can leave your body in 3 weeks, which was wrong. It only takes three days for the bulk to get out and two weeks to disappear from your bloodstream completely. The information that I acquired was false, but it helped somehow to set up my mindset in a positive spin allowing me to get rid of nicotine from my body.

I made a subconscious commitment to myself that if I manage not to smoke for three weeks, then I would not have any reason to smoke. That is how I did. I wish I knew the information I am giving you now through these books back then, I am sure my ordeal of withdrawal symptoms on a psychological level would have been much much more serene.

The second reason which is a very real fear and probably is the cause of many people never even attempting to stop smoking. It is the fear of never smoking another cigarette in their life.

That is the fear that was the main cause that made me not succeed when I was setting dates of when to quit smoking. I am referring to situations where I told myself that I would quit smoking next morning, or next month or next week, or when I go on vacation, or when I turn 30 or new year resolutions and so on.

When the distance of your current day until the date you set as your quitting date is far, everything is fine and dandy; it is not a threading event, and it's good that you are quitting you feel good about it, you are going to quit. A week before your cessation date it gets a little bit more real, but still, it is not that threatening.

The day of the quit you will use a range of rationalizations, like the ones I identify in my book **16 Common Smoking Rationalizations Recognized, Analyzed And Ultimate Destroyed.** , to get you out of the quit.

What I did not know back then is that when someone manages to stop for at least two weeks, I managed to quit for three weeks, then we have a choice as a human being for the first time. We have a choice either to stay away from nicotine and get our health and life back gradually, or we go back being a miserable drug addict risking our life with every puff we take.

Another thing that I did not know and also would have helped me with my last successful quit was that you do not have to think long term of what is going to happen in a month or a year from now without a cig. The secret is, and this is not just with nicotine addiction but with every addiction is to focus on the moment that you want to smoke, acknowledge that you want to smoke, do not discard the crave, recognize it accept it and then proceed not to smoke! You need to be smarter than the addiction not stronger.

Focus on dealing with every single crave or withdrawal symptoms at present do not think ahead at all. Deal it man to man to use a traditional basketball tactic.

One of the fears that make people not even considering quitting smoking is because they think that they manage stress with it resulting in not be able to imagine their life without it. The reality of the matter is that cigarette smoking and stress management have nothing to do with each other except the fact that stress causes the body to get rid of nicotine faster. The way it does that it is because stress makes your urine acidic. Our body takes the first alkaloid that finds in the blood that is nicotine and sends it to the urine to impose an alkaline effect on it. This action results in a sudden nicotine depletion from the body resulting in withdrawal symptoms, and the smoker needs to go fuel the nicotine level of his bloodstream and brain, namely to take his fix like a "real" addict he is.

The real reason people afraid of quitting is they believe to their core that they can not survive without smoking. I had the same fear for as many years I was a heavy smoker. I have the failed attempts and also attempts that I never even start as proof. The strong emotional and psychological associations we created over the year with cigarettes saturated our thoughts. We conditioned ourselves that we cannot do anything without a cig. We cannot have coffee without a cig, get up from bed without having that first cig, use the toilet without smoking, talk on the phone without smoking, having a drink without tobacco use, going out with friends and not smoking. All these associations are so much ingrained and intertwined with our way of thinking that when we decide to quit we believe that we are leaving something valuable behind, we believe and feel that we are leaving a friend like we are letting someone down! We feel a void in our chest because we feel again that we are giving up on something important.

The reality of the matter is that we do not leave anything valuable or important behind, we are not letting down a friend or leaving behind something that gave us pleasure. What we are leaving behind is a DRUG addiction which has the ability with every puff you take to send you to your grave (the lucky ones) give you emphysema not be able to breathe you will be in pain trying to breathe or have a heart attack, stroke or lung cancer!

You are not leaving anything behind, you are getting your life back, you are reclaiming your freedom from nicotine, you are escaping the nicotine prison, and you are starting your life again, the day you quit is the day that you are reborn.

Most people are afraid that the first days of quitting smoking where they might I repeat they might have severe withdrawal symptoms that those symptoms will last forever, trust me I know they will not. With each passing day without smoking, the withdrawal symptoms are going to vanish, and you will see with your own eyes and feel with all of your senses that there is a better life without smoking. You can do anything and everything you used to do with a cig in your hand but now without using one. You can have a smoke-free life, I have been doing it since 2009, and it is the best years of my life thus far. I was literally reborn, and I want you to understand that quitting smoking is not impossible at all, everyone can do it. This is shown in the numbers, we have more ex-smokers than smokers right now worldwide, and that tells me that quitting smoking is not as hard as it is presented in the media and other venues.

How to deal with the fear of failure

Everybody is afraid of something or someone. When I first started my quit attempts I was oblivious to any concern. The reason I was not scared of anything it is because I was ignorant, yes ignorance makes you fearless. The least you know the least afraid you are because you are not aware of the dangers, the more you know, the more afraid and concern you become because you are more conscious of the hazards and the possible future impacts might have on you.

Ignorance is not bliss as I said numerous times in my articles and books, and in the situation of smoking ignorance is DEATH!

After several failed attempts at quitting smoking, I realized on a subconscious level at first that I was not fighting just a stupid bad habit but an entirely different kind of animal.

Yes, I got afraid that I will never be able to stop smoking, I was desperate, and I was depressed about it. If there was a magic switch that every smoker could flip and suddenly will be free from nicotine, then all the smokers would flip that switch on a heartbeat. I know I would, I am confident about it.

After the failed attempts I tried to quit using the so-called NRT's (Nicotine Replacement Therapies) like chewing gum, nicotine patch. That did not end well, and it made me even more afraid because these products are advertised by the Pharmaceutical companies as "Therapies" There is nothing therapeutic about them at all the only thing they achieve to keep you under the nicotine influence, without breaking the addiction.

So now I was frightened, several failed cold turkey attempts left their scars on my psyche, and I reached to the point that I convinced myself that I could not quit smoking.

How I managed to overcome my fears was a personal commitment to stop tobacco use and to spear ahead until the urge to smoke would go away.

Now as an ex-smoker since 2009, now I know, and I see how ridiculous my past fears were. I understand of course that people that are contemplating to quit now the fear of failure are very real, but I want you to know that quitting is not impossible. All these concerns you have now will go away once you start educating yourself on what smoking is and also how to quit which I presented in my second chapter of this book.

Smoking is a way to deliver a highly and deadly addictive substance into your body; you need to understand that even if you do not like the sound of it. I am repeating it because that is how important it is for you to succeed in this endeavor of removing nicotine from your system, that you are a drug addict, a junkie, your drug is nicotine you need to acknowledge that to your psyche core.

You will never eradicate the nicotine receptors they are always there with you, but you can stop taking nicotine, thus remaining asymptotic from the nicotine addiction.

I am a drug addict in recovery until I die, I am a junkie that is on its drug, and as long I stay away from nicotine then I am ok, I am like people that never smoked before. I will be asymptotic I will not have urges or the unnatural need to smoke.

You need to understand that you need to remind yourself every day that if you take one puff, that can turn you into a full-blown smoker again (nicotine addict) with all the adverse effects that bring (sudden death and many other).

Nothing works, I tried everything, I am still a smoker.

I cannot say that I tried everything out there that offers the possibility of smoking.

I did try to cut down cigarettes; I tried nicotine patch, I tried a few times to go cold turkey, I decided to quit after being sick with the flu for a few days.

Did not try hypnosis I was afraid that is something might go wrong you never know what the other person can program into your head even at an unconscious level. Did not tried acupuncture the thought of all those needles put me away.

Chewing gum I did not use because I was never a fan of chewing gum, neither sprays or pills or electronic cigarette, back then it was not invented still yet, or it was its infant stages.

Most people that express the sentiment that I tried everything to quit but nothing works for me usually tried one of the above methods except going cold turkey which is literally what cold turkey means, stop smoking!

They set up their self's to fail by practicing methods that are not going to help them at all. My opinion the only method with the highest rate of success in quitting smoking is going cold turkey!

Well, Andreas someone will say you just stated that you had failed attempts using this method so how can you advocate it. Well you are right I did have failed attempts using cold turkey, and the only reason that I was failing is that I was not aware that I was fighting or I was trying to get away from a drug addiction and not a silly bad habit as I thought back then.

Years later when I somehow accepted that and researched about nicotine, I managed to break free from nicotine using the cold turkey method.

I am writing these lines because I want to help people understand that quitting smoking is possible and it is even more possible with cold turkey method, just stop smoking cigarettes.

Are you ready for Freedom?

Freedom such a beautiful word, everybody loves freedom, it gives you the opportunity to do whatever you want, whatever you like, whatever you wish and desire and nobody or nothing will be in your way.
It would be nice to be able to watch a 2-hour movie without itching to go outside to take a cig every 20 to 30 minutes (half-life of nicotine in the body)

It would be nice to be able to work for 2 and 3 hours straight without having to stop for smoking every 30 to 45 minutes.

It would be good to be able to run up and down playing with your kids without having to stop every 30 to 45 minutes to smoke.

It would be nice to be able to drive for hours without risking your life and the lives of other if you did not have to smoke every 30 minutes.

Smoking is not freedom. Smoking is your jailer and nicotine is your prison. Every time you light a cigarette you are letting your jailer incarcerate you even deeper into your own private secret nicotine prison.

My question to you is, are you ready for Freedom? Have you catch yourself wondering what would it be like not to wake up in the morning without a cough, or talk to people and see them not cover their mouth and nose because of your bad smelly breath. Have you ever thought what you could have done with all that money you are wasting buying cigs, going for luxurious vacations, buy a new car, renovate your kitchen? Do something nice for your parents, do something wonderful for your kids, buy the misses or the hubby something amazing.

Quitting smoking is not impossible, you need to understand two significant aspects of the quit. First, there is the physiological aspect; you need to remove the nicotine that floats through your bloodstream and the sooner you do it, the better. The only method that will do that safely and efficiently is going cold turkey if you want to quit smoking then you need to stop smoking, and that is what going cold turkey means. The second aspect of the quit procedure is that you need to be 100% commit to quitting smoking and 100% commit quitting cold turkey.

No backup quitting smoking methods.

If you go to a quit cold clinic or you decide to stop using the same approach on your own, then you need to go into this procedure without having a backup plan for quitting smoking. If you go into a cessation situation either clinic or on your own having an alternative plan of stopping quitting, then you are not committing yourself 100%, and with the first tiniest difficulty you will encounter on your cold turkey program, you will find an escape route to your backup plan.

Do not enter a smoking cessation program having another alternative backup up plans, commit 100% to the cold turkey philosophy and practice, it does work that's how I stop smoking, and I am smoke-free and free from Nicotine since 2009.

I remembered that on my successful quit back in 2009 I was so determined and so focus, and in the back of my mind, I was it is all or nothing this time. I prepared myself not to allow it to fail because I said to myself that if you do not quit now you will never will, and I did not really want that for me. I did not want to give myself the security blanket that it offers it was all or nothing, and I went for all. You need to realize that if you want to quit you are fighting for your LIFE, so you better make a serious commitment, 100% using cold turkey and I promise you will have more possibilities of actually breaking free nicotine than any other method.

Thank goodness you are hooked!

I do mention a lot in my articles and my books that it only takes one puff to go back to full blown smoking. Well, I need, to be honest with you some people do not get hooked with only one puff. Some of them to get away with it. Statistics say a 10%.

The difference between a person that took a puff and returned to his previous smoking regime and someone that took a puff and did not get hooked *is the realization of what he has done.*

Please let me explain. An ex-smoker that took a puff and became a smoker again. If in the future managed to quit again this person will have this previous experience (took a puff) as a lesson learned that there is only one way to stay nicotine free and that is never to take another puff again in your life. Of course, they can quit smoking again if they have the time, the chances of losing their life from smoking-related issues is significant. In a sense these people are the lucky ones, if they manage to quit again, they have a solid chance never to smoke ever again because they learned their lesson.

The other category of people that got away with it with a puff or smoking one or two cigarettes are the ones that did not learn anything from their experience. Worse in the back of their mind they think if they got away with it once, they could do it again

84

and again, they do not realize how dangerously are gambling with their lives. They will smoke in the future one or two cigarettes thinking if they get away it once they can do it all the time.

At some point, they will become chain smokers, and if they manage to quit at some point, they will always have the notion on their head that they can smoke again and get away with it. Many people are what I call yo-yo smoker, they quit they stay away from a few days, weeks months even years, and then they go back again, and they repeat the same procedure.

If they do not go back to that moment when they first took that puff and recognized what their mistake was, they will always assume that they can get away from smoking without getting hooked. Of course, this is a false assumption and are doomed to repeat this yo-yo situation.

I know what I am talking about. Two months after I stopped smoking I took a puff to see if I was in the clear with smoking, big mistake and stupid of course. I was justified back then, I was ignorant, which is not an excuse, but I thought smoking was a bad habit. I did not return to smoking that puff did not hook me up and for the last eight years maybe it gave me a false impression that I can get away with smoking.

I know that is not true and also I make sure I remind myself that every day that one puff can make me a drug addict again and I do not; want that for me anymore.

I recognize now that the puff I took had the potential to bring me back to chain smoking and this time I might not have the time to quit smoking because it would have killed me!

Stop comparing your quit smoking attempts with other's

Every person is unique as I wrote so many times in my articles on my blog and my books. I usually mention that we are like snowflakes, you will not find two snowflakes that are the same.

Asking other people on how they felt during their quit is not going to help you at all, it might give you an idea of how they did it and what they went through, but your quit is going to be entirely different, similar but completely different.

Even your past failed quits are different with each other, I remember that my former quits were different, the first attempt was with the nicotine patch. That failure made me realize a few things about nicotine, the other attempts were cold turkey ones, and in each of them, the reasons I failed was different as were the conditions and the states of my mind.

Me saying what I felt or what I did, might give you an idea of what I went through, that does not mean you will have the same symptoms as me. Every person is unique, it might be worse than me or milder than mine, you could use similar methods of not lighting a cigarette, but they will never be the same.

Comparing other people's quit is not going to help you because of its completely different experiences. We never know how a future quit will be like. The most important thing to remember is to commit to the last quit so you will not have to think of how a future quit will be because it will not exist.

The amount of how much cigs you smoke a day does not determine how hard you're stopping smoking will be.

My father was a heavy smoker for years. Moreover, his quit was not that difficult, I know I was there. He chews chewing gum (not nicotine ones) with a vengeance at first but he made it, and he was a smoker for 42 years, did about 30 to 40 cigs a day, so I know from first hand looking at my father situation and also from my experience.

People think quitting smoking is hard, it is not true.

As I already mentioned in this book and previous writing of mine (other books and articles) Statistics show that there are more ex-smokers on the planet now than smokers so that for me it says that quitting smoking is very doable and it is not impossible.

People are saying that they are in a subtle percentage of the range of 7% that manage to quit smoking is simply not accurate. I used to believe that too, and I say think because I did not search for it, it also gave me a sense that I accomplished something remarkable, well yes it was remarkable for me that I had the strength to quit and also the power to stay away from it all these years. The truth of the matter is that every smoker out there can stop smoking rather effortlessly using cold turkey method as long he or she makes the commitment to the long run.

Mindset: Quitting smoking is a simple decision; you need to tell your mind that you will commit to stopping. If you manage to do that, then you do not need to argue or discuss or resolve the arguments about tobacco. In primary lame words, you do not need a big reason to stop smoking, you can quit smoking because you only want to. Do what you promise to yourself to face and deal whatever the withdrawal period might bring, you will endure and go through that because you realize that being a non-smoker has long-term benefits.

How bad is Nicotine withdrawal?

I can speak from experience only, and I can talk about my last quit which was successful, and it was back in 2009. It was not that bad. I had moments that I wanted to smoke and I was agitated, sometimes I felt I was losing control, I was shaking a little bit, but I was so prepared for quitting that I did not let it overpower me or take over. I used my willpower which worked for me because I am a very stubborn man who will see things to the bitter end regardless if it's right for me or not. There is an easier way, *use your logic*, and allow yourself to be smarter than nicotine and not stronger, logic says not to smoke.

I mentioned again the tactics I used before, but I am repeating them now for you, maybe some of them you can use, and they will be helpful. I would chew on straws; I would eat or drink, I would go to my bed and hug a pillow until the urge would go away. I would do the airplane seat, I had this chair in the middle of my room, and I christen it airplane chair, and every time I would get the urge I would go and sit there, and I would pretend that I was on a plane. It really helped me because you can't smoke on the aircraft and my mind will help me with the urges.

These are some of the things I did, and I managed not to smoke for three weeks which are more than enough to get the nicotine out.

The reason so many people are afraid of quitting smoking is that they are worried so much about the withdrawal symptoms if they are going to be mild or severe. Most people are somewhere between. Even that I wrote that I had bad withdrawal symptoms I think that description as my physiological state was incorrect and erroneous I believe that it was more a representation of my psychological state. (in my Smoking chapter of my first book Thirsty for Health) My physiological withdrawal symptoms were mild.

How to stop prolonging nicotine withdrawal

I now know what smoking is. Clearly, smoking is one way too many, in particular in the age we live in, that delivers a very deadly and addictive toxin into our body, namely Nicotine.

Many people still think, what I thought years ago that smoking is just a bad habit and easy to get rid off. I tried to quit smoking with that mindset and did not succeed because I was not addressing the problem to each core, I was not a person indulging in a bad habit, I was a drug addict with all that comes with the term. Do I like the sound of that? No of course not but unfortunately is the truth. People who smoke tobacco cigs are drug addicts; they smoke to take their fix of nicotine, they are junkies and the only difference they have with the rest of the drug addicts us that their drug is still legal to buy and sell.

Now I am not a drug addict, but as I already, mentioned a lot in this book series I am a drug addict in recovery for life. The Nicotine receptors that were first created with my very first cig years ago are there, and they will never go away, as long I do not use nicotine I am in an asymptotic state.

In the old ways, they were mostly four traditional approaches to getting your nicotine fix, cigs, pipe, chewing tobacco leaves and smoking hookah.

Now we have a range of alternative approaches to get your fix which some of them were christened "Therapies" by the pharmaceutical companies like Nicotine Chewing gum, Nicotine patch, Sprays, candies and other prescription drugs.

Other methods are the electronic cigs, vapers they call them now or vaping, where through an electronic device you inhale into your body liquid nicotine!

So now it is even more dangerous and more likely to become a nicotine addict than before, you have all these different ways of ingestion nicotine in you, and some of them sound so innocent, chewing gum for example and so on.

BIG-PHARMA made sure to convince people that quitting sucks, that quitting is not easy, that quitting is going to bring you pain or make you feel terrible, and by doing that they are selling their so-called NRT's (Nicotine Replacement Therapies), They should call them Nicotine Replacement Torture instead!

When someone is an addict, we are not just talking about nicotine now, but any kind of user who wants to achieve detoxification. To achieve detoxification, to clean her blood and body from the substance, she must stop administrating the addictive substance into her body and not continue receiving the addictive substance using other ways. She must stop using the addictive substance forever. Take for example the alcohol addicts, Cocaine addicts, Heroin addicts, Meth addicts these people stay away from the substance that makes them be addicts to clean themselves.

Why on earth does the same principle does not apply on smoking? If you want to quit smoking, you want to stop using nicotine not using nicotine with other methods.

Cold turkey is the only method proven throughout the years to be the most efficient and the one that does not prolong the withdrawal symptoms, in 3 days you are off and in two weeks nicotine is completely out of your system

All the other so-called NRT's are just prolonging the withdrawal symptoms, make you feel bad and worse of all make you quit on your quit and go back to smoking because you find it difficult to do this prolong cutting down and also thinking that it will be like this for the rest of your life. Both of them are not true.

When will I stop wanting a cigarette

There is no period there is only experience on the matter. Every person is unique and that time will vary for each and everyone.

I was lucky because I was always a bit of a hermit and didn't and still don't have many friends. I did not have the wild or intense social life other people have. I am introvert and that in retrospect make me quitting smoking easier because I had fewer opportunities to smoke when I was not in my house or at the place of my work, and also that means that I had fewer triggers on a social level after I quit smoking.

So especially with smoking the more socially active life, you have, the more difficult it is to quit because you connect more life events and aspects of your life with smoking making it seems that you cannot live without and little social activities are left undone without you smoking.

Me, on the other hand, I might be a social outcast or a social hermit if you wish but I had less social triggers to face thus making it easier for me on a mental level to stop smoking and doing stuff without a cig in my hand and mouth.

Even if you have an intense social life that doesn't mean is impossible to quit it's only a matter of retraining your brain to do those social situations without smoking.

If you relapse does not blame the method.

Relapses are not determined or defined by the method you used to quit. If you quit using NRT's and then relapse you cannot blame it on NRT's. The Same philosophy applies with cold turkey if someone used the method cold turkey to stop in the past and he or she had a relapse in the future that doesn't mean you can blame the relapse on cold turkey. The two do not have anything to do with each other; they are not dependent on each other at all. The reason you had a relapse is that you smoke a cigarette, you took a puff!

One of the oldest ways of nicotine delivery and addiction.

Oral tobacco is as addictive as cig smoking, it might not have the same nicotine absorption, but it has the same result, it turns you into a drug addict just as well with lots of dangers as smoking. Mouth cancer and bad teeth are one of them except of course all the other diseases and conditions inflicted by nicotine. I never had any inclination to chew tobacco, and it has not that I did not have the chance I think two major things played a role not to use tobacco like that.

First, when I was growing up, I would see these western movies from the 50's where cowboys were chewing tobacco, and usually, it was old men with yellow brownish mustaches and with missing teeth. That was not a pretty side, so I was repulsive by that and second I knew that girls did not like men that chew tobacco and let's face it you do want to increase your chances of being liked by girls and not the opposite.

Let's celebrate with a Cigar.

I described an episode two months after I quit smoking where I took a cig from my cousin and took a puff to see if I was still hooked or was still able to enjoy it. The cig was nasty and was smelly, and I almost throw up.

My mistake was that even that I knew on an unconscious level that nicotine was the addictive agent consciously I was still

92

considering smoking as a bad habit. I was under the false impression because I stop for two months I had it under control. Luckily I did not relapse, and that is why I said instead of celebrating my successful quit every April I will do it the end of June from now on because even for the briefest of times I did relapse when I took that puff, not a full blown one but at least a tiny one. I now know that a puff can take me back to smoking because it is not a habit but a deadly addiction. (put the photo of the cake and the cig with the big ex above here)

There is a real danger that ex-smokers face after months or years without nicotine, and that is to forget why they quit smoking. They think by having a puff or a couple of cigs or a cigar to celebrate after all those years without smoking that they can keep in under control.

The sad and sometimes deadly truth is that you lost your quit by doing that and you are in a procedure of returning to be a full-blown smoker with all the adverse effects of it.

I smoke whenever I want, I have it under control.

In 2009 I stopped smoking successfully, and I learned from an excellent friend of mine a few years after I quit that he also quit smoking and I was so excited because he is one of my best friend and naturally I want what is best for him. Recently we went out for lunch, and with great disappointment, I saw him lighting a cigarette after he finished his meal, and when I told him that I thought you quit smoking he said yes, but I have it under control he said I smoke occasionally and on weekends. I have it under control he repeated, and it sounded more like trying to convince himself than informing me about his smoking.

You need to understand and I know to some of my readers out there it seems that I am repeating myself, but this is important to comprehend. Smoking used to be along with chewing and pipe the most modern ways of delivering nicotine into your body; now you have NRT's, electronic cig, hooka's, and much more. Unfortunately, my friend is going to return gradually to his former full-blown smoking.

Smoking creates a nicotine addiction one of the deadliest mankind has ever experienced. You do not control a highly addictive drug like nicotine is, it controls you.

Now I admire and respect my friend he is a very resourceful and smart man and if I did not know the things I know about smoking I might have fallen into the same trap as him. Thinking that having a couple of cigs now and then will not make me an addict again that I can control it.

Many ex-smokers falls into this trap; they see other friends of them or people that worked together going back to smoking and giving the excuse that they have it under control and they start smoking too thinking that they will control it too.

The reality of the matter is that ex-smokers that lost their quit tend to minimize the degree of their relapsing smoking because that is how they justify it, they are in denial, and they are doing again what we're always doing, they rationalize illogical arguments to allow themselves to continue smoking.

If for a moment can stop the rationalizations and see what they are doing to themselves then they will want to quit.

Can you relapse from second-hand smoke?

Second-hand smoke was one of the major issues I am sorry about because while I was a smoker and at some point a chain smoker I exposed many people to my second-hand smoke of my cigs especially my lovely mother which I love so much.

I did ask her forgiveness for my second-hand smoke with I was polluting the house for so many years and she forgive me, I only hope I did not cause her a health issue with that.

You cannot get a relapse from second-hand smoking if you are an ex-smoker, that doesn't; mean you should not avoid it.

Nicotine when is coming in contact with air it dissipates. What second-hand smoke has though is 4000 chemicals that are also not good for us and are poisonous, like carbon monoxide and hydrogen cyanide among others. The bottom line is second-hand smoke is not going to make you go back to smoking, and it's smart to stay away from it. It is full of poisons; it is like standing above a burning fire inhaling the smoke or inhaling the fumes that come out a car exhaust.

Were you addicted to Nicotine?

That is an unusual question, and in some way, it might describe the whole smoking situation for me.

This issue for me makes me understand and clarifies in my head a range of aspects about smoking.

First, when I was a smoker for 16 years I was not harboring a bad habit I was a full-blown junkie, and my drug was Nicotine. Yes, I was a drug addict, and yes I was addicted. Am I proud of it? No, of course, I don't think anybody likes to be addicted or hooked or controlled by anything either man or woman or substance because if you allow yourself that then you surrender your freedom and yourself to other people or situations. You let your life and your actions be controlled by others or in the case of smoking you allow a chemical a very deadly and addictive chemical to rule your life.

Nicotine tells you when to go to smoke, and the chemicals don't care if you are in a crucial meeting or in the middle of an important event, or your kids want to play.

It controls your life, and you are responsible for that with that first puff you took out of a cig years or months or even days ago.

So yes I feel ashamed that I allowed myself to be a drug addict for 16 years! Wasted my health away my money away, lost personal and professional opportunities because of smoking and at the end, I did not have anything to show for.

That is the first thing I realize and also helped me understand even more of what I was doing to myself day in and day out, slowly killing myself poisoning myself intoxicating myself and for WHAT? I am infuriated with myself honestly of how stupid I was all those years.

The important thing is even if you have regrets and this is a big one is I wished never to light that first cigarette so many years ago. I am one of the lucky ones since the year 2009 I am smoke-free, I don't have any major health issues, but you never know, you never know what smoking for 16 years did to me. Every day for sixteen years I was inserted in my body 4000 chemicals and toxins which about 80 of them are scientifically proven to be carcinogenic in nature! You never know what they did to me or what will do to me if they find the right ground to develop.

Every day I wake up, and I thank myself for having the desire the strength and the opportunity to quit smoking back in 2009.

I will never go back to smoking not because I forgot how it was to be a smoker, honestly sometimes I catch myself not even thinking about it which is good and bad at the same time.

It is good that it does not bother me, the thought of me smoking looks for me something of a science fiction movie with things that do not exist anymore, I feel that my smoking was like an evil fairy tale that never happens to me.

The sad thing is that as human beings we tend to remember only the good moments of our life's and forget and throw to the deepest places of our subconscious the painful and dangerous memories. Hey, it is a defense mechanism of the brain to keep us sane and functional.

This defense mechanism or your brain is literally a trap for ex-smokers like me; we only remember the so-called "safe" cigs. I know there is nothing good in a cig now, so sometimes in a moment of weakness and forgetfulness of why you stop smoking in the first place, you take a puff from a cig a friend gave you or a cigar to celebrate the birth of a child, another thing I find so much oxymoron. Why do guys celebrate the bringing of a new vibrant life into this world with a practice like a cigar smoking, that only brings death and destruction to the smoker?

Lots of reasons, stupidity, ignorance, social upbringing, and much more, I had them all, I was stupid for 16 years, I was ignorant for 16 years, and I was on automatic pilot trying to live how society wanted me to live and not how I wanted to live.

I will never smoke again because I know now what smoking is, is one of the many delivery methods of putting into your body a deadly addictive toxin, namely, nicotine into your blood.

I also know that I will not smoke anymore because I remind myself that I am going to be for the rest of my life a former drug addict. Who will not have any symptoms of wanting a cig if I never take another puff, because that is what it needs for me to go back to full blown smoking, tiny small puff!

Another thing that showed me that I was addicted was the sheer volume of how many cigs I was doing a day! You realize an addiction when you smoke 40 to 80 cigs a day at some point in your life

I know I will quit again

Many people including me at some phase of my life used this argument to postpone quitting smoking or justify a failed quit. Yeah, I have time to stop again… do we? really? Have time? To quit again?

Smoking kills 50%! of people that become regular smokers, and that is not a very favorable possibility, I do not know about you, but I only have one life, and I want my odds to be in my favor.

My advice that emanates from my experience is this. If you decided to quit smoking try to realize the following before you begin your quit:

1. Admit to yourself that you are a drug addict and that you are fighting a deadly addiction, make yourself aware that you are going to fight a drug dependency, not a bad "habit." You are a drug addict; your drug is nicotine, it does not matter that nicotine is legal to buy and sell that has nothing to do with the fact that is a deadly addictive toxin. It has you under her total influence. Understand that by quitting smoking you will break that control

away by stopping tobacco use and the most successful way to do that is to stop putting any more nicotine into your body.

2. Understand and realize that you need to be 100% committed to the quit, you will not give yourself the chance to have a backup plan as an alternative way of quitting smoking. Cold turkey method is your only way, do not allow yourself to have security blankets and backup plans that will make you light a cig and fail your quit. Be smart, make a firm decision not to smoke another cigarette anymore for the rest of your natural life.

3. Realize that you might not have the desire again to quit smoking. You might not have the strength to try again and the most fearful of all one, you might not have the opportunity to quit again because you had a heart attack or a stroke or lung cancer or even worse than death an emphysema that will cripple and devalue the quality of your life forever.

4. Do not assume that all the bad things of smoking will happen to someone else the odds are against you quit now and reclaim your life. Away from any addictive, deadly substances like nicotine is, it is in your hand to take control of your life and remove the power that nicotine has on you.

I smoke because it gives pleasure or because I like it or-or-or

I used to use this rationalization as an excuse and as an argument when others were asking me. I was honest in my reply, do not think I was lying or pretending, I thought that I was smoking because it was genuinely thinking I was getting pleasure.

Now, of course, I know the sad truth, which is the fact I was a drug addict, sure it is not illegal to get it it is everywhere, in every other corner you will find a convenient shop that sells them, but that does not make it any less of a deadly drug.

I thought that by feeding my drug addiction I was feeling pleasure and it is easy for someone to understand why in my addictive mind it was perceived like that.

When I would go into withdrawal, I was feeling sick, unhappy miserable, itchy, angry, irritated and then I will smoke, and all these negative and unhappy feelings will go away. I would feel much better a euphoria would take over me, and I had the false impression I was giving pleasure to myself.

The reality is that I was feeding my addiction and maintaining the nicotine blood level so they do not drop below the levels that would make me feel the negative withdrawal symptoms.

Pleasure is not something that kills you from inside out, makes you look older and waste your money down the drain!

One of the many things I realized after I quit of course was that from the 30 to 40 cigs I was doing every day for the last two years of my "smoking" career I was only "enjoying" about five maybe six cigs out of 40. The rest were not giving me any "pleasure" may be that subconsciously help me understand even more that it was not pleasuring I was getting but feeding a dependency that was controlling me offering me nothing what so ever.

I will probably enjoy the first cig I will smoke right after I wake up and it is understandable because while sleeping you do not get any cigs no nicotine enters your body and you are at the top withdrawal level so yes you enjoy that cigarette because you are feeding and replenishing your depleted nicotine blood levels.

Other times were when I had coffee because nicotine and caffeine do interact each other on a chemical level. Actually, nicotine inhibits the caffeine absorption that's why smokers drink more coffee than they really need.

After meals, those cigs were seemed to me to be enjoyable. Sometimes after having sex and of course with alcohol!

The sad fact is that even if in my mind I had divided my cigs to "good, " and bad cigs ALL of them were killing me, and ALL of them are killing you.

At some point in my life I was not breathing enough I was not breathing well, the incident that made me see how bad cigs were was the event that I almost fell after running a small hill to deliver one of the computers I fixed to a client.

That is when I realized that breathing is more important than smoking! I know I was stupid, ignorant and in denial.

Stop torturing yourself by quitting with gradual withdrawal

It is the way my brother is trying to quit smoking the last time I talked to him, and I did not say anything because I did not want to hurt his feelings that this method is one of the methods with the least success rate.

People cut down cigarettes in the hope that eventually they will get rid of their nicotine addiction. It does not work like that. Sure if you are smoking let's say 20 cigs a day you are a one pack smoker and you start reducing the number of cigs you are smoking. In the beginning, you are ok. Unfortunately when you reach 6 to 8 cigs a day and you are basically taking only 40% of your nicotine requirements that's when it starts to get difficult. I tried that in the past by replacing my 3 to 4 packs a day with rolling cigs, I thought that if I had to roll my cigs, I would end up smoking fewer cigs a day and in time I would be able to unhook myself from them.

Big mistake I end up sitting on the weekend and rolling all the cigs that I needed to smoke during the week!

This way of quitting smoking is the worst that you can think of, and it has the same principle as NRT's. The theory behind NRT's is that you start introducing into your body the nicotine quantity that you approximately get with smoking on a daily basis and gradually reducing the amount of the nicotine gum or the nicotine patch until in theory will be more easy for you to quit.

Many things, in theory, work 100% and are perfect this is one of them. In practice, it 's a bad idea. You are setting yourself to fail by putting your body into a daily and permanent drug withdrawal; you are extending the withdrawal period for days and sometimes months.

On the other hand, cold turkey only asks you to ensure a 72 hours withdrawal period window, and sometimes it is not that bad as you expect it to be.

If you hate someone, you should tell him to smoke a cigarette every three days that would make him be on constant withdrawal state something that trusts me is not fun to be in. Talking as a drug addict in recovery for the rest of my natural life withdrawal symptoms should be as quick as possible and cold turkey method is the only one that offers just that. Cold Turkey method is like when you have a wound, and you must remove the bandage, you do it in a continuous swift motion, you don't remove it slowly causing pain.

Cutting down cigs or using vipers or electronic cigs or various NRT's "solutions" only prolong the withdrawal process makes you psychologically weak and end up going back to full-blown smoking. These techniques are excellent in theory, but in reality, they do not; work because we are dealing with addiction here not some simple problem that its solved with gradual withdrawal.

Have one puff it's not a big of a deal.

Every journey starts with a small step. Not all trips are good for us, some of them are indeed beneficial, and we reap positive information, and some of them are lousy, and they destroy us either physically or emotionally or both!

In a journey there is a beginning and an end, all things on this planet work like this, we get born, we live our life's, and then we die. It's life's algorithm.

The first time a man or a woman has a sip of alcohol there is a 10% chance that person will turn into an alcoholic, it will turn into an addiction that in the end might cost them their lives.

If that person quits drinking alcohol then in order not to relapse back to be an alcoholic, they should never take another sip in their life again. If they do, they will reintroduce the addictive substance (alcohol) into their blood and have a significant possibility of becoming a full-blown alcoholic again with all the disadvantages that come with it.

Same thing applies for heroin and cocaine addicts, and the same principle applies for ex-heroin addicts and ex-cocaine addicts.

The one thing that baffles me until today, so many years after the surgeon general of USA in 1964 came out and announced that smoking is an effective way of delivering a deadly addictive toxin into our blood namely Nicotine people still today do not see it as an addiction but as a bad habit.

That is the first mistake we do; we do not; recognize smoking as it is which is a very efficient delivery method of a deadly substance namely nicotine.

Smoking cigarettes is a dangerous addiction and are the same as alcoholism, being a heroin junkie, being a cocaine junkie, meth addict, and many similar toxic dependencies.

The reason smoking is not perceived even until today as a drug addiction it is because of three primary reasons.

First, it is not illegal to buy cigs; it is everywhere and readily available to consume. Not being illegal like the other drugs makes people lose focus of its deadly addictive ability.

Second, for years, they were commercials on television promoting it along with other products like milk, meat, cheese, chips and sodas and so on. The consumer in his mind made the assumption that cigs are just another consumer option he has and not a deadly poison.

The third reason for years everybody in the movies smoked, you saw actors like Humphrey Bogart and other well-known actors and actresses smoking. People imitate other people and especially people that they admire and like. Smoking through the movies was passed like something adults do, making the youth wanting to try so that they will become adults too, they made it look smart and sophisticated, people smoked because they thought it made them look more stylish and more modern and so on.

The sad truth is and excuses my French all these are a bullshit promotion strategy orchestrated by the tobacco companies to hook as many people on nicotine so that they will make money! I know it sounds tragic and inhuman, but that's the truth.

Like every journey that starts with a small step, smoking starts with a puff, just a puff. Never forget though that the difference with other journeys is that there is a 50% chance your smoking journey will end up in you dropping dead. I do not know about you but I know I have only one life and 50 – 50 chances are not the odds I want to play my life with so if you are an ex-smoker or a non-smoker and thinking one puff will not do you any harm, I urge you to reconsider.

Go out there and ask chain smokers and smokers or relapse smoker how come they smoke again, you will see the majority of them will say in remorse that one day they just took a puff.

So I relapsed it's only natural.

Unfortunately, big pharma lobbying and promotion and advertising tactics have as a result government agencies to be influenced so severely that they advise people through official documents not to worry if they slip during a quit, that relapsing is something natural and to be expected!

What a huge pile of s@it, excuse my French! The people that are trying to quit are fighting for their LIFE; they are trying to get rid of deadly toxins out of their system so they can reclaim their health and the quality of life they had before becoming smokers and there is this ridiculous advice from government organizations? Where they supposedly care about people's health?

I am wondering if they gave the same advice to alcoholics that try to quit or heroin addicts or cocaine addicts, why don't they have the same "helpful" guidelines they give for quitting smoking?

I tell you why because two out of three drugs I mentioned are illegal that is why and alcohol is not as addictive as smoking is.

I am repeating that when someone drinks alcohol for the first time, there is a 10% he will end up having an addiction to alcohol. Smoking Is an entirely different story, when someone smokes for the first time 90% of the people get hooked on nicotine, that's how strong nicotine is, but we give the smokers that are trying to quit a window to escape their quit. When they hear from so-called specialists that you need to take NRT's and that if you relapse a few times, it is a natural way of quitting then you are not helping them you are giving them an excuse to fail!

I bet all these specialists never smoked in their life; they do not know what it means to be under the influence of a powerful and deadly drug like nicotine is.

Well, I may not know much about everything else, but I do know a few things about addiction, I was a nicotine addict for 16 years, and since 2009 I am a recovering drug addict, and I will be as long as I do not; take a single puff from a burning cig.

I tried most of these other methods, and I failed because they are not dealing with the cause they are treating the symptoms. The cause of my addiction was the administration of nicotine in my body through cigs, NRT's and other so-called "therapies " they just treat the symptoms the withdrawal symptoms. The bottom line is that they are just another replacement for the delivery method namely cigs, you are still a nicotine addict, but you are not smoking anymore, that's not a solution.

The way I quit smoking and manage to get rid of the addiction was cold turkey, just stop putting them in your mouth and commit to yourself that you never light another cig in your life that's how you quit smoking!

106

Of course, all these so-called specialists are probably funded or have strong ties with big-pharma. Big-Pharma sends them to little trips now and then, get a commission every time they sell their products, supply their office equipment the list of biased ties and decision-making is endless. Check the link for further information on how to find out if your doctor received payments and why. https://projects.propublica.org/docdollars/

 I dare you to go and ask ten ex-smokers how they quit smoking, and I bet you 9 out of 10 they will say cold turkey, and I mean people that are ex-smoker more than a year.

Smoking a cig while on a quit is not a natural thing to happen, having a cig while trying to quit is a natural thing to happen when you relapse not when you are quitting.

Past successful quits is a beautification of failure.

Previous successful quits is an oxymoron, if you were smoke-free for two years and then you took a cig, then you did not have a successful quit you just lost your quit, and that my friends are not a success, it's a big fat failure. A successful quit is a quit that you will take it to your grave, you stopped smoking and never smoked until you die from natural causes now that's what I call a successful quit!

Now people when they fail they always try to blame others for their failure or try to minimize the effect of their actions. The classic example is when we were in high school if we wrote well on a test or an exam we will always say I got an A or I got A+. If we did not go well for a test or exam we got a C or D we would say he or she (meaning the teacher) gave me a C or gave me D like it is not our fault. It is immature human nature to acknowledge and accept success and reject and blame others or other situation for our failures.

Same thing with failing at a quit, instead of recognizing the reason that we failed on our quit which was smoking a cigarette we baptize our inability as a "successful quit." Makes the blow easier on us it protects us from admitting that we failed, their kind of beautification of our language does not help us grow as human beings do not help us learn from our mistakes so that we will not repeat them in the future. Using "beautiful" words to disguise situations is presented in a fabulous humoristic way by George Carlin, check out this video.

That is why you see people having a series of so-called "successful quits" which in reality is a succession of failures and the lack of evaluating them and looking at them as such denied them the opportunity to have a final successful quit.

The sad and dangerous aspect of viewing failed to quit attempts as such is that smoking is not chewing gum you might not have a next chance or opportunity to stop because the odds are against you with every added cig you smoke. One day you might drop dead because you failed to learn from your previous failed quit smoking attempts.

I will die a smoker if I relapse.

In my many failed cold turkey attempts yes I had many failed attempts at quitting smoking using cold turkey that doesn't mean cold turkey is not the best method to stop smoking it just means I was doing it wrong. One of the fundamental mistakes, as I mentioned before, I was doing was the fact that I did not know what I was facing and dealing with, in the back of my mind I was under the impression that smoking is a bad habit and I will get rid of it like that.

A lot of the times I would say to myself that if I do not manage to quit now, I will probably smoke until smoking kills me. I knew smoking kills, and that is why I wanted to stop so I will not be in danger of dying from lung cancer, back then I had no idea that more than a significant percentage of the smokers that die are dead because of nicotine and not because of lung cancer. Smokers die mostly from cardiovascular diseases like heart attack, stroke, and much more.

Next time you decide to quit be more committed to your quit because if you failed and you lose the quit, then there is a big chance you will never find the strength, desire or even worst the opportunity to stop again.

Did I learn anything from relapsing?

As I already mentioned numerous times before, I had a lot of failed attempts at quitting smoking. The question I am asking myself today since 2009 after my thus far successful quit is this, Did I learned anything every time I had a relapse on nicotine with my previous tries?

I did a soul-searching on this question because I wanted to find the truth not so much for me but for all those people out there, who want to quit and help them with this information, some of you are reading these lines.

I cannot honestly say that I learned anything every time I was relapsing back to nicotine because if I did, then I would have stopped earlier, that is my conclusion. The doubts and my ignorance made me search deeper of why I cannot quit; it forced me to look into more of what smoking is.

It forced me to find out about nicotine and even back then didn't understand its addictive powers I started getting an idea of what smoking is and that is not a bad habit as I initially thought in my head.

My failed attempts and relapsing made me question the very nature of smoking which enabled me gradually to reach a level of awareness of what smoking is that allowed me to better prepare for my last thus far successful quit which lasts since 2009 and I intend to keep it for the rest of my natural life.

I am wiser now than when I was a four pack a day tobacco smoker, I have more respect for myself and the people around me, and I realized to my core that smoking is not healthy at all, plus I saved much money since I quit smoking.

You better think of your health first and then think the money too is that something that you want to do for the rest of your short life on this earth? Which is going to be even shorter if you continue smoking?

Just be smarter and wiser from nicotine not stronger.

If I quit smoking, I will be nervous all the time.

The reason smokers fear this is because they assume that smoking helps them manage their stress.

I am going to say this again, managing stress and smoking have nothing to do with each other except that stress causes rapid nicotine removal from the brain by urine acidification. Alcohol also has the same effect; you drink alcohol your urine becomes acidic the body takes the nicotine from your body and throws it to the urine to alkalize it. Quick rapid depletion of nicotine occurs the smoker enters in a withdrawal situation, smokers they need to smoke to replace the lost nicotine and at the same time assume that smokers are managing and dealing with stress. In reality, the smokers satisfy their addiction and get their fix.

I used to have that fear too that after quitting smoking I would not be able to control my temper or my nerves or my stress because deep in my mind I thought that it was helping me. After several quit smoking attempts and living and experiencing the withdrawal symptoms, I believed that those bad feelings and unpleasant situations would carry on for the rest of my life.

The reality is that they will go away you might have some rough time the first three days, I repeat you might, and then you will see that everything that you were afraid was not real they are not real it is in your head. Once the nicotine is out of your system, then you need to retrain your brain to live without a cig and face every social situation you had as a smoker without a cig.

It is a learning procedure nobody can show you exactly how to do it, but you can make it if you make a commitment never to put another cigarette in your mouth.

Common symptoms after you quit smoking.

They are called common because mostly they appear to a big percentage of the people that quit smoking, saying that that does not mean every person that quit smoking is going to feel them or experience them all.

That is not to say that if you did not feel them that you were not addicted to nicotine. How easy or hard it was to quit smoking has nothing to do with a very real physiological drug addiction like nicotine creates in your body.

One of the many symptoms I experience when I quit smoking and in particular the first month was that my appetite became larger I was eating more and more frequently.

I knew from other former smokers, and from info, I read online that it is something that too is anticipated, but nobody explained why this is happening. My own simple and of course ignorant explanation was that because I do not have something to do with my hands and my mouth I replaced it with food!

It is years later and more accurate when I started reading information that helped me understand that nicotine forces our sugar storage in the liver to be released into the blood just in 7 seconds! This way smoking provides energy to your brain faster.

If we wanted to have the same effect with food, it would take 20 minutes from the time we ate something until the glucose the natural sugar that it is the fuel of our brain to reach the brain.

I was eating way too much because I was replacing the calories that the powerful surge of sugar I was getting because of the effect the nicotine had on my liver.

One good way to make sure you will not have these cravings and also you will not feel light headed is to drink natural juice often. It will help keep your blood sugar level in a relatively stable situation without feeling any significant severe cravings.

It is a good idea to keep this juicing regime for the first three days to give the body the chance to start healing itself and recalculating and finding the natural way of regulating its sugar levels again.

Years of forcing your liver to release glucose and fat into your bloodstream messed the usual procedure up, it needs some time to learn to retrain itself to regulate the sugar levels without the aid of nicotine induce function.

Getting sick after quitting smoking

When you stop smoking is the best thing you ever did for your health. So many people get the flu or get a cold after they quit tobacco use, and they blame it on quitting smoking! I know it is crazy. You know what else is crazy, you used to waste your hard earned money buying a legal drug that offers you nothing, I could mention all the stuff nicotine and carbon monoxide does, but it is pretty clear by now how deadly and poisonous smoking is.

As you put more time under your belt away from smoking your immune system will become stronger, and you will see that you will not get colds or flu that often.

Your lungs cilia will start to work again, and they will start cleaning your lungs from all that toxins and the tar that was accumulated of mindless smoking all of over the years.

Coughing after quitting smoking.

They cough because the cleaning mechanism of their lungs and their immune system is getting healthier, and with coughing, they start to remove all those toxins accumulated in the lungs and all over the body. For some people, their coughing is very intense, and lots of them think that they have lung cancer. The majority of the cases are simply the body is using coughing to remove the poisons in your lungs forcibly.

If you spit blood, then that is another story you should see a doctor that's another scenario altogether. Even if you do not spit blood and you are coughing hard that interferes with your life then see a doctor check the symptoms out.

I did some minor coughing after I quit but not very severe, it lasted for about two months for me, for some, it might be fewer, for others, it might be more in duration. Depends on the person and the situation, how many years you were smoking, how many cigs you smoke a day and other factors.

Tell everyone you know that you quit smoking

I decided to stop with my dad. It was back in 2009 while we were coming back from the city. I told him that I would quit smoking, and to my surprise, he said let's quit together.

When my father said that I felt magnificent, I was not going to do this alone somehow. I felt secure and safe, and I think that I would have the support of my father give me the emotional and psychological strength to succeed.

Of course like Joel Spitzer says, and I agree with him because the guy knows a lot about smoking cessation is to quit for yourself and no one else. Because if the other person or situation you are quitting for does something that will make you angry at them or disappointed, then you will start smoking again because you are not quitting for you but for them.

I think though that with me and my father I was not quitting for my dad, I was quitting for me, I told him I was quitting so he will know and in the back of my mind that would keep me accountable for my actions after that day. Also, I told my mother, and I do not think to anyone else.

By telling my parents that I was quitting smoking as I said I was keeping myself accountable. If they saw me smoke after the fact that I told them I stopped then I am sure I would feel a failure and ashamed and I did not really want to feel or be in a situation like that so for me telling them was something that would help me quit with more success.

The fact that my father also wanted to quit too was a bonus because I would not have to see him smoke while I was on my quit procedure! I think that would make my quit effort harder.

I now know that I should have told more people because in the back of my mind I was like if I failed its ok only my parents knew so nobody would make me feel ashamed or show them I am weak.

So yes telling as much people that you will quit is a must and is a huge emotional boost for your psychological ego and health and better prepares you for the quit ahead.

Also having the support of friends and family will make the transition more pleasant and easier. I am confident now that if my father were not quitting at the same time as me, it would be much harder for me to stop smoking, especially since I was living with my parents at the time under the same roof.

Having a support group of friends and family is an added arrow in your quiver in your effort to quit smoking. When you feel you want to light a cig, you can always call a family member or a friend and talk it out especially the first three days. They can come over to you, or you can go to them.

People will reward you with verbal support or give you gifts for quitting. The most important thing of all you should reward yourself at the end of every day you had without smoking even if it is a pad on your back.

Do not keep cigarettes near you.

With all my failed attempts and with my last successful one since 2009 I always got rid of my cigs from the house, also ashtrays, matches, lighters, tobacco rolling machines, anything and everything that had anything to do with smoking.

The reason was that if I wanted to smoke let's say 10 p.m., and there were no cigs in the house. To have a cig, I would have had to dress up get out of the house get to the car drive to a convenience store buy cigs then come home sit on my couch and smoke.

All the events that I described take time and in my case from having the urge to smoke until coming back with cigs in my hands that would have taken me about 30 minutes.

In those 30 minutes is more than enough time to rethink my decision, resist my urges, change my mind, persuade myself out of smoking. If I had the cigs at home then that 30-minute time window for me, other is fewer others is more, wouldn't exist and I would not have a chance to talk myself out of smoking.

That is the reason you need to destroy all of your cigs and disappear anything that can help you smoke easy, and in your comfort zone, you need that time to get your senses back and your goal which is quitting smoking back on track.

Another reason people keep a pack of cigs on them or have cigs at home is that they think that by having them on them or stashed in the house are being stronger than the cigs.

That is not a good idea at all because, in a substance level, Nicotine will kick your butt every time, that is how you got hooked in the first place, you took a puff you introduced Nicotine into your body you got addicted, and you started smoking.

By keeping cigs on you or in the house does not prove you are stronger than nicotine, it only increases your chances of smoking again because if you want to smoke its right there in the reach of your pocket or the draw of your desk. The crucial time that you gain if you did not have them on sight is gone no time to talk yourself out of it!

Also when I was a smoker, and I am sure many smokers had the same incident, many times. I will drink my coffee light a cig, and then I will put the cig in the ashtray and do something else come back drink some coffee and light a cig and after I light it realizing that I have not finished the first one which is still smoking in the ashtray!

If you have cigs on you, you actually can light a cig without even consciously be aware you did it and then your quit is out the window.

Practical Tips to kill and deal the urge to smoke.

If you are reading these tips, it means only one thing. It means that you decided to stop smoking. Something inside you clicked and made you see what are you doing to yourself with smoking. You don't like what you have become (a Nicotine Addict), and you made a commitment never to smoke again, to never be a slave to the nicotine prison.
The following tips are practical things you can apply when the urge to smoke comes knocking on your door.
A lot of them I also use a lot of them I didn't. You are unique, you are a snowflake as I often say in my books. You need to practice with these tips and adopt the ones that work best for you.

You need to remember that the desire to smoke usually is more frequently present when we are experiencing one or a combination of H.A.L.T. (Hungry, Angry, Lonely, Tired)

Tip Number 1

Quit smoking using the Cold Turkey Method. It is the Method I used back in 2009 to stop, and it's the method with the highest success rate. If you don't believe me, ask 10 people that quit smoking more than a year. I bet 9 out of 10 quit using cold Turkey method.
So why even bother with other methods, choose the winning one.

Tip Number 2

Do not carry cigarettes is a no-brainer. If you carry cigs with you, it's like being an alcoholic that goes to a detoxification clinic but has with him a bottle of alcohol. Get rid of the cigs. They are the delivery method of nicotine into your body.

Tip Number 3

Many pharmaceutical companies present quitting Cold Turkey as something impossible because. They argue that quitting like that it's not helpful for the smoker and that gradually reducing nicotine is a better quitting practice.

Excuse my French, but that's bullshit. Many smokers cannot pass the idea that they will never smoke again, that's why NRT's (Nicotine Replacement Therapies) area so popular. The secret is to focus on one day at a time. Concentrate and commit to going through your current day without smoking. Do not concern yourself about tomorrow the day after tomorrow a week or a year from now. That's not your fight, that's not your goal. Your goal is to get through the day without smoking. It is a doable goal, it's not overpowering, and it's achievable.

Tip Number 4

The years or smoking have created pretty strong associations. Associations that you cannot live without smoking. For a lot of years, you smoked when you were happy or sad. Fearful or stressed. Every emotion and every action of your everyday life you associate with smoking.

No wonder when you decide to quit you feel like you abandon a friend like you are abandoning something that is beneficial for you.

You need to stop thinking like that, you need to stop rationalizing a deadly addiction like nicotine is as your friend.

You need to change your mindset that you are escaping a terrible prison, you need to set your mind in a status that you are not leaving anything good behind but only death, addiction, and deception.

You need to get the red pill as Neo did in the Matrix movie, you my friend need to wake up from the fog of the nicotine trap.

You are not depriving yourself nothing by stopping smoking that's the attitude you need to adopt if you want to be victorious.

Tip Number 5

You should be proud that you are not smoking. You are entering a better state of awareness and in a new life that it will only get better from now on. When you reach the bottom the only way to go is up.

Tip Number 6

Urges will occur at any moment. The secret is to go with your life as you used to while you were a smoker. Do not change anything. You need to start retraining your mind that you can do anything and everything you used to do as smoker but now as a non-smoker.

If some social functions or events are hard to resist and you feel you will smoke if you attend then do not attend. Skip them for now especially in the beginning. You can always do them later when you have more days under your belt as a non-smoker, and your self-esteem and self-confidence is much higher.

Tip Number 7

You decided to quit smoking for some reasons. You should sit down and write them all on a piece of paper. Keep that piece of paper where you usually kept your cigs. Have it with you always, and every time you feel that you want to smoke get that piece of paper out and start reading it really slowly. Use that list like your prayer.

Whenever you feel weak, and you feel you are going crazy or you think a cig will solve your problems use that list as a way to talk with the God you believe in.

Tip Number 8

When you were, a smoker have you ever had a cig after you had a fresh, natural juice? Think about it? Did you? The answer is probably no. The first three days which are crucial drink lots of natural, unprocessed juices. Juices have high levels of Vitamin C which helps your body getting rid of Nicotine faster. Also, the glucose in the Juices will help your body bring back to normal levels your blood sugar.

Tip Number 9

One of the mistakes I did after I quit smoking was to use food as a crutch. I end up gaining another 22 pounds. To avoid that make sure you eat smaller meals at least 6 times in a day. By doing that you will never feel very hungry and you will not gain much weight.

Also, another way to make sure you will not gain any weight and at the same time aid, you in getting a better health status is exercising. The best exercising is walking. Start with five minutes a day and work your way up until 45 minutes a day.

Prepare healthy snacks like fruit salads, and veggie salads. Nuts. Stay away from processed and full of white sugar products. When you are hungry, you can always snack on your snacks.

Tip Number 10

The illusion that smoking helps with stress and anxiety is a deadly one. You need to understand that smoking only feeds your addiction and nothing more. It does not help you cope with tragic events of your life. It does not allow you to ease the blow when the crisis hit your life.

You need to remember and comprehend that smoking is not the solution, on the contrary, it will disable you and not allow you to deal the situation efficiently and productively.

Tip Number 11

When you see an ex-alcoholic reaching for an alcoholic beverage, you know that there is a big chance he will become alcoholic again. That's the mindset you should have for your nicotine addiction. It only needs on the puff, and you are a smoker again. I mean think about it. That's how you got hooked in the first place. You took a PUFF! So no matter how long you be off smoking days, months years decades remember this, you only need a puff to go back.

Tip number 12

When the urge comes, do not try to will power it out. Stop and think, acknowledge it and then take the logical step of not smoking. Do not try to be stronger than nicotine is smarter.

Also, remind yourself that smoking is death. If you smoke, it will kill you eventually. So if you want to die prematurely, then I guess smoking is for you. I have a feeling though that you are a smart human being.

Tip Number 13

There are people in other countries of the world that are very poor. Sociological studies have shown that many times parents that are also smokers will not buy food for their kids instead they will buy cigs for them!

Now you may not be that poor but think of all the money you threw down the drain all those years, killing yourself from inside out. Making the Tobacco companies richer and stronger economically and politically.

From the first day, you quit smoking get a big glass jar and start putting the money you were going to use to buy cigs in it. A glass jar because I want you to see the money every day you were literally throwing away. At the end of your first week open that jar and count that money. You be surprised. Now get that money and buy something for a change that will not kill you.

If you don't want to spend them in a week and want to keep going even better, more money for you in the future.

Tip number 14

If you think about it we can live without food for a lot of days, we can live without water for 3 to 7 days, but we can't live without air.

Our breathing is what synchronizes and balances our homeostatic status of our body.

We take it for granted because we are not consciously ordering our body to do it, it's an involuntary procedure.

When starting to feel a void and your stomach starts to ache, and sweats of anxiety begin to take over your body you know that the urge to smoke is knocking on your door.

When you feel that awful emotion that emotion that cripples your movement and makes your head spin that's when you should use the next technique.

Close your eyes and center yourself, relax, inhale as much air your lungs can take. Count in your mind until four or more if you wish really slow and then exhale slowly. You might get a bit dizzy, so it's best to sit before you do this. Continue until you find your balance, until the panic effects ware off until you stop feeling suffocating. Do this until the urge to smoke is not there anymore.

Deep breathing exercises are your first line of defense against the urge to smoke. You can do it anywhere, at any time. It is your secret weapon, and the best is it doesn't cost you nothing!

Tip number 15

In 2009 I attempted my successful quit. I name it successfully because I haven't smoked since yet. One of the things I would do was the Airplane seat. Let me elaborate. When you are on a plane traveling smoking is not allowed. So what I did was I took a chair, and I christen it airplane chair.

Every time I would have an urge I would take a book and sit on the airplane chair. I always read while in the plane and guess what else I wasn't doing. Yep, I wasn't smoking. So I would sit there reading my book pretending that I was traveling on a beautiful tropical island. I sat there until the urge was gone.

You can use the same trick as me. Maybe you would listen to music from your iPod or watch a movie on your tablet or read from your tablet or if you are an old nerd like me read a real book!

That's something you can do in comfort in your house, but what happens when you are out of the house. Well at the beginning I advise you to go to places like movie theatres that smoking is not allowed, you can go to museums, reading libraries, you can go to non-smoking places (bars, restaurants clubs) they do exist just search for them. Do you stay indoors, go out and live your life smokelessly, prove to yourself that you can do it. Raise that self-esteem and self-confidence up. Crash that depression you might feel that you are losing out on something. You are not, you are fighting for your life and do not no one derail you from your commitment.

Tip Number 16

When I quit in 2009, it was only 4 years after I come back from Greece. I immediately immersed myself in work, I was doing 3 to 4 jobs. I will wake up 5 a.m. and sleep midnight every day for 4 years! As you can imagine this time of timetable did not allow the opportunity for me to develop a social circle outside my jobs.

So when I decided to quit back in 2009, I told my parents about it and maybe a few good friends I still have until today. By doing that I kept my self-accountable and responsible. I raised the bar of not failing even higher. People know now that I was going to quit so if they saw me with a cig in my hand then I would disappoint them and also I would feel that I let them down.

What it doesn't mind is your social circle is one or thousands tell people that you are quitting. I will make your commitment to quit even stronger. Remember you are quitting for you, not for anyone else but not letting people down and not being ridiculed because you failed is a powerful emotional and psychological weapon that will help you be victorious with your quit attempt.

Tip number 17

Another thing I did when I was quitting was to chew on drinking straws while I had the urge. I would take a straw and cut it into 3 to 4 pieces, and I would chew on them with a vengeance until the desire dissipates. My father used chewing gums (not nicotine ones) Whenever he wanted to smoke he would chew on them. It worked for him. I remember he did that for about 6 months and then he stops.

Tip number 18

Drink cold water. After you drink cold water, the urge to smoke goes away. Drink as many as needed.

Tip number 19

Brush your teeth with mint toothpaste, brush them slowly, enjoy the flavor of mint in your mouth, you will see that the urge to smoke will go away.

Tip number 20

Put a rubber band around your wrist, whenever you think of smoking pull that rubber band and release it on your wrist. Yes, it's going o be painful, and that's the whole point. For years you associate smoking with pleasurable activities. Like drinking coffee, eating food, having an alcoholic beverage, making love, having the illusion that you are distressing yourself and so on.

Now with the rubber band, we need to associate smoking with a not pleasant feeling with is a pain, whenever you feel like smoking use that rubber band in time you will see that the urge to smoke will go away.

Tip number 21

Go for a walk or do some exercises. If you can't go for a walk, you can always do some yoga exercises or some light weight lifting exercises. Check with your doctor if you can do that.

By doing an activity while you are in the mood for the smoke, you are refocusing your mind somewhere else, and that will help you forget about it faster and easier. There are hundreds of athletic activities you can do both inside your house and outside. Search them choose the one that fits your requirements.

Tip number 22

Take a cold shower. That I promise you will make you forget of any desires to smoke.

If you don't want to take a cold shower, wash your face with cold water.

Tip Number 23

Call a friend of a relative and ask how he or she is doing. Chat with them as long as it takes until the addiction urges wares off. You can ask a few friends and family members to be your support group. Tell them that you are quitting smoking and if they can be your phone buddy while having urges.

Tip Number 24

You can talk on the phone with a cessation counselor or experts for free. The internet is full of people that are more than willing to help you out in your time of need. And the good thing is it's free, and it's 24/7 available.

Tip Number 25

One of my favorites and I used it a lot. I am still using it for other areas of my life until today. Keep a diary. In it note the time that an urge emerged. Write how you felt. Write how much time it took to dissipate. Write what did you do to kill it.

Remember to see your watch the moment it starts and also after it goes away. When we are in withdrawal area, we mostly overestimate the time that urge took to come and go. This will give you a more realistic view of your condition and prove to you that is not that hard to win your freedom from nicotine.

Chapter 4
Second & Third Day Of Your Freedom

Second day towards your freedom.

The second day of my quit was not something that was new for me; I had failed attempts to quit before that lasted at least four days so I was let's say somewhat experienced and prepared for the events that might happen. The difference between my earlier quits and this quit was that this time I made a commitment, I was really into it, I was determined not to let anything and anyone and above all myself to interfere with my effort of getting rid of smoking.

If you are quitting for the first time or you had failed attempts in the past, and you are in your second day congratulations, do not let anything or anyone or even yourself to ruin this. All the people that successfully stop smoking they had the first day without smoking a second day without smoking a third day without smoking and so on. You are at the very beginning of your journey that will set you free from the prison of nicotine. Always remind yourself that you are a drug addict getting rid of your drug, the nicotine and as long you do not use you be asymptomatic to the addiction, you be free from the chuckles of smoking and all of its health dangers.

Pat yourself on the back for being without a cig for a day it is not a small thing. All great tasks are done with that first small step, and you should be proud of yourself. Stay the course do not give up, apply the same things you did the first 24 hours for the next 24 hours, and you are on the right track for success.

Do as you did the first day. Deal and face individually every time you had an urge to smoke, acknowledge it, don't fight it but do not give into it also. Recognize it and then chose to ignore it, do something else, occupy your mind and your body with something more healthy or useful.

If you stopped on a Tuesday then your second day is Wednesday, a workday for most, you are in a better position and situation now because you have the experience of a day behind you. You managed to be smoke-free for a day. It might not feel like is a big deal but trust me when I say this to you, IT IS! Embrace your success. Now you have a road mad for the second day. Now you know what to do if you get an urge, you have the algorithm for success that works for you. Your first successful smoke-free day is a valuable lesson and experience that you should use to help you go through the second day.

Be smarter than nicotine not stronger remember that.

Symptoms of quitting smoking

The only sure thing that is definite about quitting smoking is that there is a physiological withdrawal period of 72 hours, that is when the physical symptoms occur and peak. After that initial 72 hours, the urges or the withdrawal feelings the ex-smoker feels are mostly psychological and are also caused by minor physiologically adjustments the body makes learning how to function and work normal again. Learning how to work without nicotine inside it disrupting its normal functions.

All the other symptoms that different people have, some are common yes they share a particular pattern but others they are unique to their host, and it does not mean you will have them too. You might not have any symptoms at all, or you may have hard symptoms, that is the whole argument I am trying to make, do not postpone or cancel your quit because you saw or heard other people describing horrible stories of severe withdrawal symptoms.

130

I remember I had different withdrawal symptoms in my previous attempts at quitting; each failed quit I had different withdrawal symptoms and with various severity levels characterizing each of them.

So the bottom line is your quit will have different withdrawal symptoms, you might have mild ones or none! Alternatively, you might have hard or excruciating ones, you never know until you try and when you come face to face with them, then remember that you make a substantial commitment to getting rid of your smoking that keeps you a prisoner to the nicotine trap and addiction.

What is going on with our Blood sugar?

I am an amateur runner; I started running back in April of 2010 after I gain 22 pounds because I stop smoking the year before (2009) and the reason I started running was to lose the weight.

I lost some weight, and at that period, I was triumphal about my weight loss. My competitive bug bit me, and instead of focusing on losing more weight I shift my attention instead on running faster and longer in my races.

One of the things I used to do and still do if I have the time is to always train at a higher altitude of where the race will be held, and I always try to train at least twice the competition altitude. For example, if my race is at the height of 420 meters then I will work and train at 800 meters.

A lot of you will ask why? Why would you do that? Well, the higher I go, the less oxygen I get, by training on higher altitude I train my lungs to optimize and utilize less oxygen so when I go in a race competition that is held in lower altitude, I can achieve more because my lungs will use more oxygen thus increasing my performance.

Anyway, what all this have to do with smoking? Well, our brain to function correctly needs two things, glucose (natural sugar) and oxygen.

The first time I started training at high altitude, I would get disoriented and dizzy couldn't focus well because I did not get enough oxygen and until I get into shape I had those symptoms.

When you stop smoking one of the many symptoms you might feel are headaches, difficult to consecrate, disorientation, time perception. You might don't remember what you did 5 minutes ago or one minute ago.

Now, this is happening because for many years nicotine was bullying your liver into releasing glycogen and fat into your bloodstream tricking your brain that you are, now you know why when you smoked your appetite was disappearing, you were getting sugar and fat through the liver and this action happened in seconds!

Now that you quit the sugar and fat that you were getting with that unnatural way must be provided the good old fashion way, you have to eat or drink those calories. That is why is a splendid idea to drink natural fresh squeezed juices for at least the first three days it will help you with the stabilization of your blood level and help you avoid all the unwanted symptoms I just mentioned earlier.

So if you get any symptoms like that, it is because you are not getting enough calories, drink your juices and try to divide your calorie intake evenly during the day. Have some breakfast, lunch, and dinner, try to distribute your calories during your time evenly.

Do not fall into the trap and the false conclusion that you will have this symptom forever, give time to your body to remember how to function again normally without a deadly toxin telling it what and what not to do.

Like for me, it took time for my body to adapt to the high altitude less oxygen supply same thing applies to you too, you need to give some time for your body to adjust to the new situation.

What's wrong with my coffee?

When I was 31 years old, I was diagnosed with a stomach and duodenum ulcer. It was awful, the diameter of the wounds inside my stomach was 1 cm each! I would sit down to eat, and as soon the first bite of food entered my stomach I would run like crazy to the toilet having severe cases of diarrhea! It was appalling to me both physically and mostly emotionally. This chronic disease made me afraid going out and socialize because of the fear or not having a toilet nearby, even today after all my healthy lifestyle psychological remnants of that way of thinking still occur if I go to a public place the first thing I want to know where it is the restroom!

The good doctor informed me that I need to stop using coffee and caffeinated drinks and also quit smoking. It turns out smoking destroy the inner layer of our stomach, and of course, coffee is an irritant and causes the stomach to produce more acid resulting in more damage to the inner layer of the stomach and the existent wounds.

With real drug addict attitude, I responded I would give up coffee, but I cannot give up smoking! Like I was bargaining a tv set or a new car! Anyway, I did manage to cut coffee; I did it gradually and also stop drinking colas that were full of caffeine too.

Now this sickness of mine, stomach ulcer a bad thing on its own helped me bust the myth that a smoker cannot live without his coffee. I did it for four years, and I saw firsthand that hey I could smoke without drinking coffee, so that subconsciously planted a little information that later on, I want to believe, helped me realize that if you stopped caffeine consumption, you could do the same with nicotine.

Stop drinking coffee has a positive effect on me when I finally decided to quit smoking. I did not have that notion that if I quit smoking, I will never enjoy my coffee ever again. For me, that issue did not exist so in a manner of speaking that helped me with my quit easier let's say because I had one thing less to worry about.

Now saying that caffeine-like nicotine is a drug, they both have addictive nature, I give you that caffeine in small quantities in research have shown to have beneficial attributes but nicotine had none useful characteristics, it is pure poison and its killing you from inside out like most of the cancers do!

Also, nicotine interferes with the metabolism and absorption of caffeine from the body, an example to clarify it even more. When you smoke, and you drink coffee, the amount of caffeine that the body manages to absorb is significantly less than the original quantity you receive, and that is because nicotine is interfering with the caffeine absorption.

Now that you stop smoking, and if you are a coffee drinker, and you continue to keep drinking the same amount of coffee you might notice some changes on your mood. Pay attention, the thing that I am going to say doesn't apply to anyone. If you felt agitated, on edge and wired that's because the lack of nicotine is allowing your body to receive and absorb more caffeine quantities that you used to take. Now not all people might feel this effects but if you feel edgy and irritated try reducing your amount of caffeine daily input.

For example, if you are drinking 4 cups of coffee every day, try reducing it to 3 cups a day for a week to see how you feel, if you still have these unpleasant feelings of edginess and irritability reduce it to 2 cups a daily try it for a week and see what happens.

My advice is to stop drinking coffee altogether you do not need it to stay awake. If you increase your fruit and vegetable consumption overall and start exercising even 30 minutes of brisk walking every other day, you will see that your energy levels will go up and you will not have to use stimulants like caffeine to get you through the day.

Plus, caffeine stresses your adrenal glands and in time fatigue crawls in because your energy levels are depleted, and that is the days you feel like you were hit by a bus. What you usually do is to wait some days for the adrenal glands to recuperate so you can start "bullying" them again with caffeine.

Also, your poor liver is working overtime to remove caffeine from your body being a drug as it is.

You need to understand that smoking is not a rational act to do, nicotine and the other 3999 chemicals you put in your body destroy you from the inside out, and there is nothing ordinary about that.

Now that you stop smoking, and your body is starting to remove all those deadly and toxic substances from your body, it needs some time for your body to return to a state that is normal, to go back to a level that was before you ever started smoking all those years ago. It will take the time to start correcting and healing, so yes be patient, let the body do its job, it knows better than you, understand that you are a drug addict, even if you don't like the term. I know now that I was a drug addict and most importantly of all I know, I will be one in recovery as long as I don't put in my body nicotine ever again.

The psychological and emotional stages of losing someone or something.

All my previous failed quits were doomed from the start for one reason or another. Writing this book is mostly about me, by saying that it does not mean I do not want to help people like you dear reader.

The primary reason though that I write this book except helping guys like you to quit smoking, of course, is to find out more about myself and try to understand what actually happened to me when I was under the pernicious influence of nicotine for 16 years!

All my former failed quits lack certain characteristics like I was ignorant, I thought smoking was a bad habit and not an addiction, I thought I knew that nicotine was addictive it did not register in a conscious and logical level. Second I was using the willpower method; I thought if I were strong enough I would manage to stop smoking, that doesn't work most of the time.

It did work for me, but that's because I am a stubborn man, so stubborn that I will lose my health to do something.

How stubborn I am, well think about the following story, when I first took a puff from a burning tobacco cigarette back in 1993 the first thing I felt was a burning sensation from my mouth down to my throat, then it was that nasty burning smell that made me want to puke my guts out.

Now those unpleasant experiences were the body's way of telling me, hey stupid stop doing that it's not good for you but me being stubborn I continued smoking until the burning sensation went away and the puking feeling disappeared.

So for me being stubborn worked but I had more going for me. I was and still am a loner, all the jobs I had were jobs carried out with no one around. So I did not have many social triggers that social smokers have when they quit smoking.

Going out for coffee was not an issue for me because I stopped drinking coffee years ago because I was diagnosed with a stomach ulcer. Going out for a drink, never drank too much alcohol, don't get me wrong I did get drunk when I was a student but generally speaking me and alcohol not the best of buddies.

Anyway, you got my meaning, that's why it worked for me. I used my willpower for a year and for a year I was always walking on hot coal as smoking was concerned. After I managed to hold for a year then all the tension and anxiety I had if I was going to return to smoking disappear. What happens was that my mind accepted the fact that I was not going to become a smoker again.

Now there is an easier way of the willpower, and that is common sense. First, you need to recognize that you are a drug addict, and once you truly get that into your head then you will be able to see that you are in a pit. The only way to stop being in that pit trap is to stop receiving nicotine either through tobacco smoking or other ways (electronic cig, vaping, nicotine gum, nicotine patch, hookah, etc.) once you realize that your escape from the deadly traps of nicotine is 100% assured. I am sure that since you are on your second day without smoking that the mindset I just described is what you identify with.

Don't try to be stronger from nicotine by using your willpower, be smarter than nicotine. When the urge to smoke comes, I repeat the mindset you must adopt. Do not fight it head first like you are a bull, recognize the fact that you want a cig and choose not to have one, do the smart thing not the stupid drug addict thing.

That's how I was wrong if instead of head budding with nicotine recognized the fact that I am more intelligent than a chemical I wouldn't have suffered all those mental agonies and stress of not smoking.

That's how I see it anyway. All the people that are successful in helping people quit smoking advocate that you should be smarter than nicotine not stronger (Alen Carr, Joel Spitzer)

Now I want to share some more personal stories with you because I feel that that's the only way for me to discover and find out more about myself and in the process maybe help you.

I decided to quit smoking, well it was more than a one way for me. At the age of 35 I had the fitness level and energy of an 80-year-old man, I know it sounds like I am exaggerating, but an 80-year-old guy could easily beat me in a 100 meters race.

Smoking really messed up my internal organs, stomach, lungs, etc.

I had my revelation moment where I actually saw myself dying around the age of 50! And I didn't want that for myself. So I stopped smoking, using the willpower, the only way I knew how and I succeeded but as I said many times in this book there is an easier way and I briefly described it earlier in the previous paragraph. Now, after I stopped and especially the first two weeks of my last successful quit which was back in 2009 I was needless to say very emotional, at the time I didn't know how to recognize the emotions I had because I was an ignorant little man with the emotional capacity of a wasp! But now that I know I realized and recognized that I went through distinct emotional states that if you are quitting you need to be aware.

First two weeks because I was using the willpower method which you should not use, and because I was ignorant I was in a state of fluctuation as my emotions were a concern. Pondering back now I distinctly remember falling from emotional situations or don't want to quit when I was arguing with myself that I have to quit then I would get desperate and I would whimper that   I can't stop smoking. All these thoughts were always occupying my head, and sometimes it drove me crazy, I was irritant and could not focus not so much from the physical withdrawal of nicotine but because I was quitting using a method that did not really address the problem that I was a drug addict.

Denial state

Anyway, even if I was quitting using my common sense thoughts of denial and actions of isolation will happen to you too. It's only natural to experience these emotions because down

139

deep in the twisted sick mind of a drug addict quitting smoking is like giving up a "friend" a loyal friend that kept us company through bad and good times, through worse and happy days. In the messed up and unsound mind of a drug addict that giving up smoking is like losing someone close and valuable, and the first stage of loss is to deny that it happens.

Except remembering these really frustrating emotions I had the unfortunate opportunity last year to experience firsthand and in a very intense way the denial and isolation that brings when I got divorced.

For the first two months approximately I couldn't believe that I was alone again that my ex-wife was not there with me, I would pretend that she went away for a trip and any moment now she will come home. Sometimes I swear that I could hear the front door of the house opening and she would walk in saying hello and ask me how my day was like she always did.

Lots of many incidents like that I could present showing the denial phase of losing something.

The first three weeks I would minimize my already minimally social interactions I had, and I think that's a good thing to do at least at the beginning of your quit. Minimize, not remove completely that's not a good tactic.

Let me give you an example, a friend of yours calls you and invites you to go out for a coffee if your friend smoke then doesn't go! Now at the beginning and for at least the first 2 weeks. If your friend doesn't smoke then by own means go. Did you get the philosophy?

One of the right tactics I did, and I can say with much certainty that it was an excellent decision on my part, was that I informed all the people that I knew that I was quitting smoking. That made me feel that I couldn't fail because if I did then I will have to accept and face all the ridicule, and judgment and disappointment of those people and that made me accountable not to break my quit. Even if you have only one friend let him, or she know.

Anger State

I said all that so you can comprehend the things I am about to say to you next. While I was on my quit process after the denial phase was over another phase kicked in, and for a period of time, I was angry with everything and everyone. I was irritant, and nothing could satisfy me.

Friends of mine will call me to see how I was doing or my mother would ask me how I was doing, and I would end up being angry with them or envy at them, or people will not call as often as I would like and I will resent them for it.

They were moments my anger was elevated to rage for no parent reason, well now I know that anger, envy, resentment, rage, and discomfort are part of an emotional phase that happens because we leave something behind either is right or wrong for your physical or emotional health

Quitting smoking is not just the physiological aspect of it, that's only 1% of the process, 99% is psychological. Leaving behind a way of living even if that way of life and acting was killing you from inside out it does create emotions that need to take their course, so you be able to heal yourself from the drug addiction.

My lack of knowledge back then made the whole procedure of escaping the nicotine prison harder than it really is. I am telling you all these things, so you will realize that quitting smoking is much easier task than nonsmokers, governments, big – pharma and anyone else claims and wants you to believe it is not.

By being able to recognize why you feel the way you feel at the moment it happens it's a powerful tool to possess and will enable you to stay away from the nicotine pit efficiently and never look back.

I went through the anger phase with my divorced; they were times I was angry with myself for doing less or doing more, I was mad at my ex-wife I called her names and so on. My anger bursts were random and not programmed, the realization that the relationship was over created all the feelings an angry person feels. When rage got hold of me, I would smash against the wall objects that we bought together, or I would resent the fact that she kept facts from me from the start of our relationship and many other things.

So yes if you are quitting, after the denial phase at some point you might get angry, and envy and resentful and have a level of discomfort that you are not accustomed to. If you have these emotions, and sometimes are going to be strong ones try and be patient and work through the waves give it some time it will pass away as the denial phase passed. If you have a friend or a family member that you can talk with when you have these emotions it will help you immensely to go forward.

After the initial two phases, denial and anger then the most dangerous phase and stage begin namely bargaining.

Bargaining State

If anyone is going to lose his or her quit is during this phase because that's when you start having these strange and twisted dialogs inside your head.

142

These dialogs usually come in moments where you are not feeling well. You be disoriented unfocused, you feel that you want to smoke a cigarette, or you have some great discomfort, and you rationalize it by saying to yourself, I will smoke only one cigarette, and then I am a good boy/girl, and I will never smoke again. You will say one cigarette won't kill me, thoughts illogical and unreasonable like the ones that you made all those years, so you will give permission to yourself to continue practicing one of the stupidest and deadliest actions a man invented, smoking tobacco cigs.

You are having thoughts like, it's ok I can smoke a few cigs now, and I can quit later. I had that kind of thoughts when I was in my quit back in 2009, that's why I had practical things to do when I had those thoughts. I knew that I shouldn't smoke so whenever I caught myself arguing with my little voice in my head pushing me to light a cig I would do some things which many of them were wrong. I would eat and drink, I would chew on straws until the urge and the bargaining thoughts go away. I will go to my bed and hug a pillow until the voices quiet down and the urge will go away, and finally, I would utilize the so-called airplane chair. I would pretend I was on a plane traveling and as you know smoking is forbidden in aircraft and I would just sit there until the urge, and the cravings will go away again.

There is a healthy list you can follow which contain the things that you can employ which will effectively kill an urge or eliminate the bargaining voices that try to make you smoke in your head. I am sure some of them you already did on your first day of your quit. Some of them I repeated in the previous book. Repetition is the mother of learning that's what I say.

Things you can do to kill an urge and stop the cravings

1. Deep breathing. This is my favorite urge killer because it's always there for you. IF you are alive, it means you are breathing, so when something triggers you to think of smoking and the craving demands a cig instead of lighting one just stop what are you doing and do deep breathing. I did not use this technique when I quit myself basically because I didn't know that existed, but now I use deep breathing whenever I feel I am stressed out or want to relax and focus. What I do is I inhale as much air as I can through my nose, count comfortably until 12 and then exhale through the mouth, I do that as many times as I need until I feel this euphoria conquering my mind and I can feel the tension is not there anymore.

   Another way to breathe which will allow you to be able to have more control and it will balance your spirit and synchronize your psyche with your body is the following. Breathe while counting in your head you until 4, then hold the air in your lungs by counting again in your head until four and finally exhale the air counting in your head until 4 again.

2. A lot of people swear by this, every time you have a thought of smoking have a rubber band around your wrist, and every time you have an idea of wanting a cigarette to pull that rubber band and let it hit your hand. Of course, you will feel a slight pain, but that's the whole idea. See for years in our sick twisted voided from logic and reason addicted mind we associate pleasurable things with smoking so now with the rubber band we are setting things straight on their right track. Smoking is not pleasurable it's deadly, smoking is not needed for you to have the pleasure and a happy life so every time you

have a pleasant thought, and it involves smoking hit your hand with that rubber band and retrain your brain of the false association.

3. Drink lots of water, when you have the urge drink lots of water or drink lots of natural fresh squeezed juices. Did you notice that when you were a smoker when you had a glass of juice or water, the urge of smoking was not there? Well, use that to your advantage now.

4. Do Calisthenics or stretching exercises or lift weights or go for a walk in a nutshell when you have the craving, move around, do not stay still, do something that will make your heart beat a little bit faster, and you will see that the urge will fade away.

5. You can brush your teeth with mint the freshness of the mint will make you feel better and take your mind away from smoking. You can use other aroma or kind of toothpaste as long as works for you.

6. Take a cold shower or take a cold and a hot shower the alternative temperature will make your mind away from smoking.

7. Call your support person or your brother, sister, family member friend and talk it out with them when you get the urge, the conversation will take your mind again away from thinking of smoking.

8. Chew on something like a sugarless chewing gum, DO NOT use a nicotine gum! We are quitting smoking, so we get rid of the nicotine in our body not replace the nicotine getting from a cig with a nicotine gum!

There are a lot of things you can do to kill an urge the first algorithm here is what I call T.T.C.U. Which is Trigger → Thought → Craving → Using you want to break this cycle, and the way you do it, in a nutshell, is this? You minimize as much as you can your social interactions at least the first 2 weeks that are not necessary for your survival. Don't go out for a coffee or for a drink or to eat with people that smoke, instead stays home this way you limit a lot of triggers. When you have two weeks under your belt, and your self-confidence is better then start socializing again and deal with the triggers one by one (man to man as they say in basketball). When you have thoughts of smoking use your rubber band, you can stop the craving with all the ways I just mentioned, and the result will be not using that deadly poisonous toxin.

In the bargaining phase of my quit, I was successful. I was not so fortunate with my divorce when you bargain you say things that you don't really mean or really do, you just say them. It gives you the false idea that everything will be ok which is not the case, in the case of my divorce I called and emailed my wife saying stuff that in my head will make her comeback. I was behaving like a kid that asked something from their parents, but they refused, and after the initial anger of rejection the child in his room starts to think new ways on how to bargain with his parents. Thinking things like maybe If I tell them to get the trash out for a week or don't watch tv for two weeks, then they will let me do the things I asked in the first place. You get the drift.

You need to remember that you are fighting for your life, that might not seem dangerous to you at the moment, and maybe people around you are not really looking at it like that, but that's the reality. If you allow your inner voices to rationalize irrational thoughts and smoke, mostly throwing away your quit, then you might not have the courage to stop in the future. You might not find the strength again to quit or even worse you might not have the time to stop again because you were diagnosed with a terminal illness because of smoking or triggered by smoking.

Depression state

After you go through the bargaining phase, then the next step is the depression stage. It's only natural that you will feel sad about the whole situation, you can't-do what you used to do when you were a smoker, and that's a good thing. In our case getting rid of a nasty addiction is a real thing, it's the psychological area you need to investigate and pay extra attention. Sit down and think really hard why and for what are you sad about and you will realize that your depressive behavior and sad feelings are not really for something that was good for you.

I mean if a loved one died or a loved one left you as it happened with my divorce then being depressed and sad about it because you will not see them again and spend time with them like you used to do is entirely justifiable and healthy for you to experience.

Now feeling depressed and sad for leaving behind a deadly addiction that robbed your health and your money for so many years is just doesn't worth it. Yes grieve, yes get depressed but do not let it drag for months it's not healthy, you must remember that you are leaving nothing of value behind both for your health and for your pocket.

Be very aware of the depression stage it's sneaky, and sometimes we don't even know that we are depressed.

That's why it's important for you to do a few things that I wished I done them when I was quitting.

Get a lot of sunshine as much as you can, go outside and let the daylight saturate you, sunlight makes you happier and also do some light walking every day as much as you can at the start and gradually aim to 30 minutes of vigorous walking every day.

Watch a comedy movie or a stand-up show, laugh. Increase your fruit and vegetable consumption.

All these activities will make you feel better than when you were a smoker, increase your serotonin levels and also make you feel better and more energetic.

Kick that depression phase fast and hard.

Acceptance State

Now that I am writing these words as my divorce is concerned I am in a transitional period, almost a year after the divorce I can feel myself escaping the depression stage and entering into the final stage which is acceptance.

What really helped me overcome the depression I had because of my divorce are all the things I mentioned above, I hope I knew their things when I was quitting back in 2009.

I can feel myself feeling, healthier both physically and emotionally, I am more centered and sure about myself, my self-esteem and self-confidence are up, and I feel ready to continue with my life.

This kind of feelings that you are going to made it with quitting cigarette I also felt too when I quit.

There was this beautiful moment of finally accepting the fact that I will be an ex-smoker for the rest of my life and I will never look back; I will never return on becoming a pitiful drug addict again.

The day you accept the fact that you won't smoke another cig in your life is a wonderful feeling, the last few months, the duration will vary from person to person, you didn't think at all about smoking. You saw people smoke, and the only feelings and emotions you had for them will be a pity.

You will see cigarette packets lying around you, and you will have no feelings what's so ever about it.

Tobacco smoke will bother you, and you will avoid it, you will not hang out with smokers and even if you do you will make them smoke outside, etc.

Acceptance is a wonderful feeling as quitting smoking is a concern. What do you prefer? To be in a position where you have all those beautiful feelings of escaping the nicotine trap or have to accept the fact that you will die in 2 months from a terminal illness that was caused by smoking because during the bargaining stage you gave in and took a puff?

I think you are an intelligent person I believe that you will continue to be smoke-free and become an ex-smoker as I am now.

I accepted the fact that I will not see my ex-wife ever again. I agreed to the fact that I will not see her in my bed every time I would wake up, I would not do all the stuff I used to do with her, we will not plan for the future, and I will never have the chance to say how much I loved her anymore.

149

I still love my ex-wife but not the kind of love two persons have for each other that plan to be together for the rest of their life and have intentions of being happy healthy and raise beautiful kids together, go through all the phases of life and grow old and grumpy together.

What are the Criteria for addiction?

Back in 1964 in the USA when the general surgeon of the country made his report that smoking is dangerous for our health, smoking was characterized as a bad habit and not an addiction. The reason he did that was that back in 1964 for something to be called an addiction it had to fulfill three criteria.

First, you must have withdrawal if you stop using it, that was in existence, and it was recognized, and it even had a name which was nicotine abstinence syndrome.

The second criteria were tolerance, the longer a group of people use a substance the more they need in time because their body is getting more efficient in removing it faster, so you need to introduce more of the substance to have the same ah effect on you.

Third criteria were an antisocial and deviant behavior to acquire the material, and that was impossible in 1964 where doctors were smokers too, and half of USA population was smokers. The surgeon general that prepared the report was himself a smoker, and he only stopped smoking a few days before the release of the report.

An antisocial behavior like stealing or threading someone to give you money so you can buy your drugs is not an issue for smoking because it's not illegal to purchase and sell.

Plus no one back then would label half the population of USA as antisocial and deviant because he or she were smoking, that's why they end up naming it a habit and not what it is, in reality, a drug addiction.

That's one of the reasons that many people back then and sadly until today assume that smoking is just a bad habit. Because tobacco cigs are legal to buy and sell, they hypothesize that the government will never allow a product that is deadly to be available!

I remember when I was in the army, and I was stationed the last two months of my tour in a secluded post. Where food water and other supplies were only available once a week and sometimes once every ten days, we would walk around the campsite looking for cigarette buds that had a few drugs on them, and we pick them off the ground and smoke them!!! Now for me, these memories clearly show that I had a severe drug addiction!

Other memories are me fishing cig buds from ashtrays when I didn't have the time or the money to buy cigs and smoked them!

Another example that showed how many addicted persons are is people that quit the first day they walk down the street, and they see cig buds down on the street, and they have this urge to pick them up! I hope if you have the same urge to control yourself!

Joel Spitzer in one of its first clinics recalls stories that were told to him by consecration camp survivors, they said that when cigs were available in the camp, they will trade food for cigs! Now if this event doesn't prove that cigs are addictive I don't know what else will. I mean think about it, Second World War two Nazi consecration camps where food most of the time was not existent and they were trading it for nicotine!

That's why it's important to destroy your cigs and remove them entirely from your life not just throw them in the garbage. I bet you anything you want when you get the urge and you know there is cigs in your garbage even if there are layers of garbage above them, you will go through that garbage like an earthworm and dig them out. So remove them completely from your life, give yourself a chance to calm down and let the urge fade away.

Another example especially in countries where starvation is a daily reality, there are people that they also trade food and even the little money they have for cigs, instead of using that food to feed their kids and themselves or use that money to buy clothes or food they are trading them for nicotine! Now if that is not antisocial behavior I don't know what is.

I don't smoke because I need to. I smoke because it's my choice I can stop whenever I want.

This mindset and this way of thinking were the ones I had when I was a smoker for sixteen years. Except for the incident that made me realize that I needed to do something about smoking. Other incidents happened during my years as a smoker. That made me think even for a brief period of time that maybe smoking is more than something I do as a choice. Maybe it's not a bad habit, and maybe it's not that easy to stop whenever I want.

When I was a university student in Greece many times it will be a weekend and I would realize late in the day usually around 10 to 11 p.m. that I am out of cigs or the cigs I have will not last me through the weekend. Usually, when that happened, I would get small panicked attacks because I didn't want to be left without cigs.

Now those small panic attacks were always making me think of why I am behaving like this? If I knew I was a drug addict then I would have known the answer, but I thought I was in control of my "bad" habit and I could quit anytime I wanted, easy breezy.

I didn't have a car back then, and on the weekend and that hour not many shops that sell cigs were open, only a few selected street kiosks were open. Where I lived, they weren't any open at that hour so they were times that I would walk in the middle of the night sometimes several kilometers to find a kiosk to buy cigs! And of course, walk back to come back in my house.

The city I was living Patra in Greece back then was a quiet city back we didn't have this Illegal immigration that overwhelms Greece and Europe today. The crime was non-existed, and I had a good life and time as a student. You could see students and women and girls walking the streets of the city during the night, and it was ok.

The thought that always popped in my mind while I was walking the streets of Patra to go get my cigs was always why am I doing this? I mean can't you stay without cigs for a weekend, I mean you are in control right? These thoughts were rational thoughts but because of the lack of the knowledge that I am a nicotine addict did not help me click to the reality of the addiction I was a slave too.

On the contrary, I will rationalize it by saying that I will go buy my cigs and on the way back I can go visit a few friends of mine that live nearby the kiosk I bought the cigs from! I wasn't thinking that maybe just maybe people might sleep or do other things and don't want a junkie knocking on their doors 11p.m. and midnight!

That's what drug addicts do and especially smokers, they are a master in rationalizing the illogical so we will get permission from our brain to continue smoking.

Another thing I would do was to call friends in the middle of the night! If they had cigs so I can go borrow some. Of course, I would only call friends and acquaintances that I knew that were smokers themselves but again, calling someone in the middle of the night asking him or her if the have cigs that today for me is antisocial behavior. Of course back then in my addicted and clouded mind was completely natural. Like I was out of sugar, and I was knocking on the neighbor's door to borrow some!

The fact that I will always make sure to have cigs stashed at my place so I won't stay without. I will always buy 3 packs a day so I will be 100% sure I won't stay without and 5 to 6 packs on a Friday just in case I don't leave the apartment during the weekend! This little incidents and practices by me showed clearly that I was a drug addict, the sad thing is that I didn't get it back then, I had to kill myself for 16 years to finally click and make the commitment to quit smoking back in 2009.

If I don't smoke while on the phone I get nervous.

When I was a student in Greece back in 1994, and also a smoker, mobile phones were not that popular yet, and they were in their infant stages of development. Every time my phone will ring, my landline, instead of running towards the phone to answer it I would first reach for my cigs if they were on me or go get my cigs first and then respond to the phone. Sometimes I will go to the other end of my apartment and then run back to answer the phone.

154

Clearly, this is not normal behavior. Now I know it's a clear sign that I had a serious addiction. What I didn't know back then but I found out while I was researching for these book series is that this behavior was not done only for me it turns out it's a bit universal. People used to run for their cigs before answering the phone.

Except for talking on the phone a plethora of other small everyday activities for a smoker they seem impossible to do if they don't smoke at the same time. This sick association is mental and is this association that you need to deal with and face in order not to smoke again.

The ridiculous fear that you cannot live without a cig because you can't manage stress without, or you can't enjoy coffee or or-or it's only in your head it's psychological, and you need to retrain your brain that you can live and enjoy your life without a cig. How do you do that? How do you retrain your life without a cig, well the best way is day by day. You don't think long-term, you face the urges (mostly mental, after the three days) one by one and you use your common sense, you outsmart the nicotine, you outsmart the addiction.

The reality of the smoker is not the same as the reality of a non-smoker, and I can see it so clearly now that because I am an ex-smoker since 2009 and I can see first hand what many smokers mean when they say that I can't live without a cig.

Of course, you can live without a cig, that's the only way you will have a healthy life, you don't need smoking to able to live your life. All the little and small everyday associations you established while smoking will fade away in time and it's in your hand as I said many times already to train your brain again to do all these little daily tasks without a cig in your hand and in your mouth.

How smoking associations occurred in our life.

How many times you saw people going by outside a church either by walking or in the bus or car, and they immediately make a cross using their right hand?

How many times we listen to an ambulance siren, and immediately we assume the worse. Ow, many times we hear the fire alarm, and we think of fire and so many other events that make our body and mind to act and think in certain ways.

One of the most famous scientists was **Ivan Petrovich Pavlov** who unfortunately is mostly known about a dog instead of his amazing achievements that won him a Nobel price in 1904.

What Pavlov noticed while working in the lab was that the dogs in the lab whenever they saw people with white coats they started salivated because they knew that soon they would get fed, so they started the digestion procedure.

This woke up the scientific curiosity of Pavlov who proceded and did several experiments with dogs that proved that there are associations between external stimuli and physical behavior.

Pavlov used a metronome which was sounded in subsequent time with food being presented to the dog in consecutive sequences, the dog would initially salivate when the food was presented. The dog would later come to associate the sound with the presentation of the food and salivate upon the presentation of that stimulus.

Something like that. Now, what this has to do with smoking. It has to do with a lot actually. The example with the phone as Joel

Spitzer explains it goes like this. It seems that at some point in my life while being a smoker I must have answered the phone and on the other side the person was chatty as hell, probably kept talking to me more than 30 minutes. Now nicotine half-life is about 20 to 30 minutes where in that time mark I must replenish my nicotine levels, but I couldn't do it because I was on the phone. I couldn't move, because it was a land line it's not like today where you have your cordless or mobile phones and if you want to smoke you just walk to your cigs while not interrupting your conversation.

So after a few of those long-winded phone conversations, I subconsciously trained myself to first get for my cigs and then answer the phone in case the phone call will be long!

I became in a sense Pavlov's dog. Now, these associations are not very common anymore. With the use of mobile phones, you can go towards the room where you have your cigs and still maintain the call, also with the caller id service now you can skip phone calls because you can call them later.

I did notice though that even when I was using a mobile phone that I would grab a cig and my lighter before I answer the phone just in case the conversation was going to turn into a stressful one.

Articles about Ivan Pavlov

http://io9.gizmodo.com/the-truth-about-pavlovs-dogs-is-pretty-disturbing-1591853321
http://www.newyorker.com/magazine/2014/11/24/drool
http://www.nobelprize.org/nobel_prizes/medicine/laureates/1904/pavlov-bio.html
http://www.biography.com/people/ivan-petrovich-pavlov-9435332
https://www.britannica.com/biography/Ivan-Pavlov

My grandfather lived to be a 100, and he was a smoker!

I hear this excuse a lot from friends that smoke and also people at work, my grandfather lived to be 90 or 100 and he smoked like a chimney, and they say it with such pride like it's an accomplishment!

People that smoke and reach ages that great means only one thing, they were predisposed to live a lot and with their smoking they managed to cut their life expectancy down! Even if that life expectancy was 10 year or even 5 years, do you know what you can do in 5 years? A lot! You can do anything you want in 5 or 10 years if you set your mind and manage your time right.

Also, these occasions are very rare, not many people have this let's call them supergenes that will enable them to live long while smoking. Also who told you that lots of years are also quality years, coughing, chest pains, spitting, getting the flu all the time, and other prone to smoking illnesses.

Longevity doesn't guarantee the quality of life and a suffering free life.

The statistics are not for the smokers, 1 out of 2 smokers will die prematurely, cutting 30 to 50 years from his life. The rest will have smoking-related conditions, situations, illnesses, and diseases that will diminish their quality of life.

Another thing that I argue with the people that boast that their grandfather lived to be a hundred and smoked is that you don't have your grandfather's DNA you have some genetics from your grandfather but not all of them! In a nutshell, you are not your grandfather! That usually makes them pause for a little and think.

158

Talk with ex-smokers that have at least one year without smoking

It is a good idea to talk to other people that stopped smoking, but your questions should be accurate and detailed, do not ask them generic questions because you will get generic answers. Generic answers will not help you make the commitment and take the decision to quit smoking or better your chances if you are already in your quit process.

Example, many people ask me if I think of smoking a cigarette and my answer to them back is yeah I am, and then I add the phrase I just thought of a cig when you asked me that question other than that I haven't thought about cigs or smoking in years now.

I don't really think about smoking anymore, and when I see smokers doing their robot mechanical movements of smoking a cig I pity them like I am sure other people pitied me when they saw me smoking prior of 2009.

Quite recently thought three incidents shook me to my core one as I mentioned before was a dream in which I smoke and I woke up so frighten that I figured I smoke for real. The second incident was at work, it was like a déjà vu moment where I saw myself wanting to smoke, and I don't know what triggers it. Maybe something that was said, a description of a situation an aroma in the air a combination of the above and that also made me feel a bit uncomfortable.

The third episode was in the car driving to work I stuck in traffic, and because I haven't driven for a long time, I use the bus now, I had to go through traffic without a cigarette, and that was another inconvenience for me.

After started watching Joel Spitzer's videos and reading his book. Also Roberts book and also Allen cars books I realized that those urges were purely psychological not real and that put my mind at ease. Secondly, it gave me an argument to set to myself the next time smoking urge might occur. This time I am able to recognize the trigger and say ah that's why I want to smoke, and that will fix it without fear of going back to smoking.

Substitutes or Crutches to Quit Smoking

It's important not to replace smoking with something else, substitute it with another alternative, usually called a crutch. When I quit smoking back in 2009 I used food as a crutch, I substituted food for nicotine, and I end up gaining another 22 pounds resulting at the age of 35 with 5.9" tall to weight about 202 kg! Yep, I was in that 4% of people who gain more than 20 pounds after quitting smoking. This happened because nobody told me or help me or show me how to deal with cravings after quitting smoking. To be fair, I didn't ask for help either of how to deal with food after I quit smoking. One of the reasons I wrote the small book "How not to gain weight after quitting smoking" and also why I am writing all of those articles on my blog. Is because I want to help people deal with the weight issue after quitting smoking.

Other people replace nicotine addiction with alcohol dependency I was lucky in that area since I don't actually hold my liquor, I get drunk really easy, and I am out fast, I got that from my mom she is the same. So drinking vast quantities of alcohol to replace nicotine was physiologically impossible for me.

Others replace smoking with exercise which is a very active and good thing to do if you are exercising for your health overall and not just to go through with the quitting process. If you are not doing it for your health but using it as a crutch to quit smoking what will you do if God forbid something happens, and you stay away from exercise? You probably go back to smoking again.

You need to exercise because you know is right for you and not as a substitution for not smoking.

It's the same example with women that once they learn they are pregnant, they stop tobacco use and after they give birth they start smoking again!!! 9 months without smoking, and as soon as they are out of the hospital they light a cig!

Crutches are temporary solutions you need permanent solutions. A permanent solution is to adopt a passionate commitment to never smoke again in your life.

Sometimes you may start a crutch and then develop a healthy lifestyle. That's what happened to me, I replaced quit smoking with food. I gain weight, and then I started running to lose weight, and in the course of just losing the weight I found my lost love for running again, and now if I don't run at least 3 times a week I feel sad and unhappy, now is a lifestyle.

Like Joel Spitzer is advocating and I completely agree with him the best useful and helpful crutch is DEEP BREATHING. It has a calming effect; you can do it anywhere anytime you want as many times you want and is always there for you, I mean if you stop breathing you die so pretty much is the best crutch to help you with quitting smoking.

After you quit a whole world of new opportunities are available for you.

When people stop smoking, they see for the first time that they can do positive changes in their life's or for their life's and they start applying it to their daily lives. People go back to college or start running as an exercise because they want to lose weight or because they want to finish their first 5k or their first marathon.

People change jobs, they try to achieve lost forgotten goals or dreams they had and so they are going for because they have this new self-boost self-esteem and self-confidence energy that derived from the fact they managed to remove from their life a deadly drug addiction.

It's amazing, but I after I quit smoking a lot of positive things happened to me except of course the health benefits I was feeling and seeing with my own eyes. I left a job that was paying less and got a better one with more money and better medical benefits.

I took a 4 months online course on how to teach English as a Foreign language. I started running to lose weight because I made the mistake of replacing smoking with food.

In the course of running, I discovered plant-based diet and lifestyle, and I couldn't be more happy about that because it enables me to retain my weight status, have an excellent running situation, and a healthy life.

So just by quitting smoking, I managed to self-improve myself as a direct result of that single thought I made back in 2009 in the car of my father as we were coming home.

You will stop thinking of smoking eventually

Yes, thinking of smoking goes away eventually. For me personally, it stopped after a couple of months since I quit smoking. The first 2 to 3 weeks for me was the most difficult, I didn't have severe episodes of withdrawal symptoms where I will shout or wanted to bring the house down because I needed to get my fix. I think it was a typical withdrawal symptom which I deal with them as they came one by one, I didn't think ahead of time, or what it might be in the future, I was really focused and concentrated on getting by the day without smoking.

I remember being in a status of confusion the first few days; my mind felt cloudy, I couldn't concentrate and focus very well, I had this constant irritation like I was on alert all the time, I remember this lasting a couple of weeks until the nicotine finally got out of my system.

All these experiences, of course, are because of the physical effects of not taking nicotine anymore, and that's great! That's excellent that's our goal to get rid of ourselves from nicotine.

So yes thoughts of smoking will dissipate in time, and you will not be bothered by the physical aspect anyway.

You will have thoughts of tobacco use in the future, and usually, you will have them every time you face a new social event that in the past you deal it or went through it as a smoker and now you are called to face it or deal with it as an ex-smoker. This thought and urges you need to remind yourself they are purely psychological triggers they are in your head, they exist because of the associations you acquired all these years of you smoking and living your life. It's only a matter of time now, and you will see as you have more time passing without tobacco use and also face new social events without smoking you will find that the psychological thoughts of smoking will fade away too, that for me took me about a year.

Because in a year you usually go through all of your natural social events of your life, and you learn and train your brain to act and react without smoking.

You will have incidents in the future more than a year without smoking which will trigger the desire to smoke, you need to remember that is not a real urge it is emotional and psychological. Use your head, be analytic, be smart and you will see its just a rare social event that you didn't face yet without smoking. Association is kicking in, nothing to be afraid of don't worry about it just let the urge slide right through you without smoking.

I also had a couple of dreams, and they were quite recent. In the dreams I was me smoking. They were so real and vivid that I woke up really confused and I actually thought I smoked for real, it was that intense, I actually thought I throw my quit away.

The reason I thought I actually through my quit away while it's obvious I did not, and it was just a dream, more correctly it was a nightmare, was that when you stop smoking one of the first items that start to work again are the physical brooms of your lungs called cilia. These brooms start to remove toxins and mucus that was accumulated over the years of mindless smoking.

Some of the mucus that comes up from the lungs contain tar. It seems that while I was dreaming that I was smoking at the same time on a physical level cilia were removing mucus from my lungs full of tar, and I could actually taste and smell the tar giving me the impression that I was actually smoking while in reality, I was not.

I am sure that I will have this kind of bad dreams again until I have tar in my lungs, my cilia will continue to clean it from my lungs. At least this time I won't get panicked, I will know that is the lungs getting better with every small piece of saturated mucus with tar removed. It will be a source of celebration, not panic and sadness.

Having a nightmare about smoking and waking up and thinking that you lost your quit it's a healthy bad dream to have, it shows that you don't consider smoking as a good thing anymore, it was a nightmare, and we have nightmares about things we don't like to happen to us again. So after I thought it over more and cooled down, I realized that I was on a good path and this nightmare was not telling me to start smoking again or that I must have wanted to smoke but it was telling me that I am in a good place away from smoking and death.

In May of 2012 if my memory serves I had a bike accident. I neglected to fix my worn out brakes of my mountain bike, and on a steep downhill route I lost control, and I end up flying parallel to with the ground for a few seconds like Superman with the difference that I didn't gracefully land like the man in the Blue and red suit!

Back then I was doing an intensive lesson in Aikido, and one of the first items you learn in this amazing martial art is to learn how to fell down, so I manage to turn my body at the last moment and get away with some bruises and minor cuts.

I picked myself up carried my bike back to the car I must have walked maybe 4 to5 km and then got my car and went to the hospital where they take care my cuts and bruises.

Why I am telling you this story, well now every time I see someone fell off a bike either in real life or on TV in the news or in movies I got the painful feelings I had when I had my bike accident years ago. I still have those feelings, and they are momentary of course they don't last as the real ones, but I can feel them.

The reality of the matter is that they are psychological pains, I associate with the falling people through my own experience I had years ago, I am not really in pain, but the mental sensations are there.

It's the same thing with smoking. After the two weeks without smoking, any desire or urge to smoke doesn't have any physiological base; it's in your mind, it's psychological like my pain is every time I see a kid fall down from his bike, it's not real thus manageable.

Every time you have an urge to smoke after quit smoking more than two weeks, should be dealt with a pause and analytic mind, it's not real, the urge is not real, do not give in non-existent urges, be smart and logical as Spock from Star Trek would suggest.

The Social Smokers

There are a few, like social drinkers. The difference is that 1 out of 10 people that try alcohol become addicted to it and end up to be alcoholics. With smoking the situation is far more dramatic and deadly, 9 out of 10 people become smokers, and they end up being nicotine drug addicts. Out of those nine people, 50% of them will die prematurely, and the rest 50% will develop a crippling disease or condition that will reduce their quality of life significantly. Smoking will kill you at the end.

People that smoke socially or get cigs from a spouse that is a smoker quit smoking harder than chain smokers. The reason is that very light or social smokers, do not have the so-called "bad cigs" in contrary with chain smokers who out of 40 or 50 cigs the ones that actually "enjoy" is maybe 5. One in the morning, one after each coffee he drinks, one after food and maybe one after having sex. All the rest he smokes without thinking their purpose is to feed and keep the addiction alive in his system. Smoking doesn't offer you anything it's a delivery method to satisfy the nicotine addiction that was created with the very first cigarette the tobacco smoker did years ago or months ago or days ago.

So for social smokers, quitting behind 3 to 5 cigs a day which they see as a treat psychologically is harder to accept and leave behind than a chain smoker of 40 cigs a day who realizes that smoking all those cigs do not offer him anything. A chain smoker will see how sick it is to smoke so many cigs and only a handful of them give him "pleasure" (in his head anyway) even those pleasurable ones are killing him too. He can see that he is smoking so much more cigs without taking anything on "return" it's easier for him to realize and get into the commitment to make the decision to quit smoking.

Starting day three of your quit

Better than the second day? Worse? Or the same?

Again you never know how bad or good is going to be, but if you had the first two days bad, it might be easier in the third. The important thing to remember here is that to focus getting through each day, and in time it will get easier, the physiological urge for nicotine will fade away.

I remember that the first days for me regarding the level of severity were as follows, bad the first day, a bit worse on the second and third day. I had a feeling of being on the plug all the time until several days passed maybe after the second week where that constant feeling of emptiness that was not getting filled went away and it was the best feeling I ever had in my life thus far.

NRT's

NRT's appear in 1994. The so-called "Nicotine Replacement Therapies" are another way of delivering nicotine into your body; they do not help you get rid of your addiction at all.

As I described in my first book Thirsty for Health in various other articles on my webpage and also in this book series, my first encounter with NRT's was when I did my first quit attempt using a nicotine patch. Back then that was the most popular I think it was in 1997 or 1998, and of course, it ends up in me starting smoking again.

In a way, I am grateful for NRT's not so much for their success rate because if you see the data is non-existent but for their failed rate which is huge.

Many people like me after trying NRT's reach quicker to the conclusion that these so-called "Therapies" are a hoax and a waste of money and do not work, me personally it helped me realized that going cold turkey was the way.

Same principles apply for the electronic cigarette, and from recent chatter and news I am reading they are trying to incorporate them as NRT's as well! Maybe by the time, these book series will be published they will. Big mistake instead of smokers you will have vapers, same addiction different means of delivery, instead of the money going to the tobacco companies they will go to the pharmaceutical companies.

A whole chapter or a series of chapters or sections should be devoted to NRT's because they are part of our life's now and also they managed to impose on society as "therapies" by the medical establishment, confusing people even more.

How to deal with people who sabotage your quit

Avoid them as much as you can, be polite as much as you can, if they continue bothering you about quitting smoking and keep offering cigs then take one and smash it in front of them, after that I don't think they will bother you again. (Nice tactic by Joel) I was lucky I didn't have any people trying to undercut my quit smoking effort and the few times people offer me to smoke I wouldn't even talk to them I would use my hands doing a jester meaning I don't want any.

Also one of my early tries of quitting when I phoned my parents and told them that I quit smoking and I am crying all the time for no reason they asked me to start smoking again. All that matters is your commitment to quit smoking because you are fighting for your life even if you don't realize it now.

Returning to normal status after quitting smoking

When I stopped smoking a few days past on, and one of the first things I noticed was that I started smelling stronger odors than I used to do. It seems that my nose began to work normal again, smoking is a nasty thing to do to your body, it dulls and saturates all of your senses with toxins and substances that a lot of them are used as pesticides! (namely nicotine) For 4 years I will get up at 5 a.m. get dressed, prepare myself to go to work and 6 a.m. I am in my car ready to drive to my workplace but after I stop smoking it was the first time I noticed the heavy aroma of my mother's jasmine that was covering the front rail of our porch. Also the seductive odors of the dawn like roses of my father's orderly pruned and situated in a straight line along the north wall of our house.

It was a shock for me and made me realize even more of how idiot I was that by smoking I would deny myself the simple pleasures of smell and the unbelievable scents that are around me.

Also, my nose could pick up odors and smells from food getting cooked; it was a feast of aromas from culinary accomplishments, something that I haven't experienced in years because my nose was blocked and obstructed by smoking, by smoke, by carbon monoxide and other deadly poisons.

For the first time, I experienced what a normal functioning sense of smell is.

Except smelling there are other important aspects of my life that I missed because of smoking, like tasting, oh my goodness the zillion flavors my taste buds were experiencing I thought I was in heaven. My taste returned, and with it, a whole new world of sensations and creation of new memories, memories that literally made me smarter, new synapses were created leading my way of thinking in directions that I never thought or felt possible.

I would sit on the table to eat, and I would make this satisfying noises with every bite I was putting in my mouth, I savor every spoonful, and my palate was having a party with the zest of new food.

For the first time in my life since I was 18 years old, I experienced and felt how food tastes like. How food should taste like, it's when I got the sense of smell and taste back that one day I cried like a little baby for realizing how stupid I was. How stupid I was that allowed myself to deny from my life these feelings, and did it on my own, I took a puff from a cigarette back in 1993 and I got hooked, I imprisoned myself to nicotine and deprived my life of having a *healthy* and happy life

Another aspect I did not handle well because I was an ignorant full was food cravings. I didn't know what nicotine does to our body metabolism. I didn't know that it forces the liver to release glycogen and fat into our blood tricking the brain into thinking that we are not hungry.

Now that nicotine was out of the scene I was hungry all the time because I didn't know that I was getting extra calories every time I was smoking. Instead of planning a healthy food program, eating many times in the day small meals and also having natural fresh juices I indulged myself in fast food, pizzas, ice tea sodas, potato chips and so on. One year after quitting smoking I gained 22 pounds and my health instead of getting better because of quitting smoking it got worse because of the overweight situation I put myself in.

When you abuse and poison your body for so many years, it needs time and knowledge to help it return to a healthy weight and to start doing its functions normally.

The overweight experience had it's good and bad, bad was that I was in serious danger more than ever for heart conditions and stroke the right news was that I started running again. I lost the pounds, and in the course of that adventure I adopted a plant-based diet which is really healthy for me and also supports my running activities (marathons, 50k trail running, etc.) fully

Also, another aspect you need to take extra attention to it is a fact of aging, when you first started smoking, you were much younger the few years you have as a reasonable person were little. You were full of energy vibrant and young, your

171

metabolism was flying, not many years after you stop smoking you are older with all the disadvantages that bring to your body needs twice as much time to repair heal or cure all that catastrophe smoking produced on it.

That's why is a good practice to start some kind of exercise, even walking a few minutes every day and gradually increasing it will help your body to clean the toxins faster, a plant-based diet also is preferable from animal products diets.

That's what I am doing since 2013, and I saw a considerable increase in my energy levels, sometimes I catch myself wishing I was living on Mars because a day there has about 40 minutes more, and I could achieve so much more with those extra forty minutes.

It will get better I promise you

The first 2 weeks without smoking were not comfortable for me but at the same time were not unbearable. I had moments where I wanted to smoke, but because I made a solemn commitment I did not cave in, I kept myself occupied until the physical urges fade away. The third week was much better than the first two, and as I was putting more distance between the first day, it got better. For me, after 6 months I wasn't even thinking about smoking. After a year that's when I started looking smokers, and I felt pity for them. I felt compassion because they are killing themselves and they are doing it with their hard earned money. Money that they can use to do a range of other healthier activities both physically and psychologically. When nicotine leaves your body, and you make sure not to reintroduce it back into your system, then it will get better.

Quitting smoking and my mental health

I had depression for sure when I was studying in Greece, maybe that's why It took 8 years to finish my studies and not 5! I was indoors a lot; I was introvert, I had anxiety attacks from nowhere. I was stressed all the time about university and work, and I think smoking for me became a self-medication item, I would drug myself, so I can feel better and also forget the many things that were "torturing" me at the time.

It's after I stop smoking that I realized that I must have had a level of organic depression because it was with me even after I ceased to smoke. This time it was more obvious because I was not drugging myself with nicotine and the symptoms of it were more obvious, my depression went away after I started running and exercising and it completely disappeared when I started eating more healthy, adopting a plant-based diet.

Now there are people out there that they are taking medication because they have mild to severe health mental issues. When they stop smoking they need to inform their doctor so the physician can calibrate the dosage of the medication to the fact that they are not smokers anymore. They even might need new drugs or no medications at all.

There are people that they can see something is not going well with them after quitting smoking because like my depression which was evident after quitting. They might notice other symptoms that fall in the mental health category and are making their life difficult or miserable or both, they need to see a doctor so they can deal with them effectively.

The bottom line is that quitting smoking is a significant step towards regaining your health back and reclaiming your life back, it's a positive step, and you should never think twice about it, just do it you have nothing to lose, literally nothing, and you have everything to gain.

Nobody knows that will gain weight after quitting smoking

That's what happened to me, and it's a reason many people do not go ahead and quit smoking because they are afraid they get fat.

Quitting smoking or quitting drinking alcohol or stopping being a heroin or a cocaine addict doesn't make you fat.

Ignorance makes you fat like I was back in 2009. I quit smoking, and I, unfortunately, replaced smoking cigs with eating. At that point in my life, I didn't care if I was going to gain weight for me. Personally, it wasn't; an issue most importantly it didn't even register as a problem or an issue that will make me back down on my decision to quit smoking.

In a lot of my articles I do say that gaining weight or not while you quit smoking should not be something to stress about, you have enough stress and anxieties while doing your quit you don't need any added stressful factor to calculate.

Well, that was me, I ended up gaining 22 pounds in a year and putting myself into other kinds of medical risks, but hey I at least removed a significant health hazard factor from my life.

I tackled the weight problem immediately once I realized how fat I was by starting running on the first phase and then adopting a plant-based diet, all described in my first book Thirsty for health and also in my other book How I lost 44 pounds using a plant-based diet.

But you don't have to make the same mistakes as I did as weight control is a concern. My advice is to go and see a nutritionist and tell him or her that you quit smoking and he or she will set you up with a nutrition diet program that will allow you to stay on your current weight and not gain any more pounds. Also, you can start exercise as much as you can under the guidance of your doctor again.

A few tips on controlling not to eat too much especially the first days is to drink lots of water lots of natural fresh juices, eat more meals small meals during the day. Start exercise as I already said. Educate yourself more about nutrition.

Medication adjustments may be necessary after smoking cessation

Smoking interferes with a lot of drugs, so if you were on medications while you were smoking now that your top smoking you need to pay your doctor a visit and let him know that your stop smoking, it might be required to reduce or increase the dosage or stop altogether, or start using another medication.

Chapter 5
Fourth, Fifth & Sixth Day Of Your Freedom

Fourth Day Without Smoking

Alen Carr calls the day he quit smoking independence day and in some level of comprehension he is right, so I am going to borrow his term for usage for this book.

The fourth day after independence day is going to be easier on you because the bulk of nicotine is out of your system and her grab on you is getting weaker and weaker with literally every second you stopped smoking.

The thing that you need to take under consideration now is that you might have more psychological urges to smoke than physical.

If the urge to smoke comes then acknowledge it and like a responsible adult, choose not to give in. Apply one or more than one of the many tips I already mentioned in the previous books to kill that urge to its root. (Click here to go to the list of the urge killers or Appendix (number) for the paperback version).

Make the right decision of not to smoke and continue with your life. Train and let your mind go through the moment without smoking. You will see that in time these psychological urges will be much easier to overcome and ignore. You will stop having them as often, and at some point, they will not even register as a problem for you anymore.

They will not be a problem anymore because unlike me you are quitting using the method of logic and reasoning, you are quitting because you recognized that you are a drug addict and you decided that you don't want to be controlled by a deadly substance like nicotine is.

I remember that as the days went by a sense of relief was taking over me, and I could literally feel myself emerging from something dark and ominous. I am sure that you are feeling much better as you read these lines. Most people describe it like a weight lifted off their chest, they actually feel lighter.

For me the way I felt like I was underwater for such long time, and now I was starting to come above the water, and everything began to become more apparent. Maybe you are having similar feelings and experiences and maybe not. The thing you must remember is that you are a snowflake, you are unique, and your quit process will be definitely different from other people. That's why it's important to keep a diary while you are quitting smoking, it will help you put your mind at ease and also help you observe the progress you are doing. A diary will keep you accountable too. To write in your diary, you have to be smoke-free so that's a motive not to smoke so you can have info and details to fill your diary with.

Joel Spitzer is one of the persons that really helped me even after 2009 where I quit smoking to understand myself better and what I used to be (a drug addict) and how to continue to be a non-smoking person.

With thousands of people cured of smoking in his cessation clinics, Joel advocates that people should quit smoking cold turkey and they should do it in their everyday life without changing nothing. I agree with that 100%.

Joel even says that there are other ways to quit smoking and he is telling that because he is a good, open-minded man. I, on the other hand, I am a bit stubborn and tend to support methods that I personally found positive results and that they are producing tangible data to work with. Now as smoking is concerned I am absolute and adamant about it, for me, there is only one way to quit tobacco use, and that is cold turkey.

Joel always started his clinics Tuesday so when the fourth day comes it will be a Friday and weekend would be on the horizon. Also by quitting Tuesday, you go through the first 3 days of withdrawal doing what you always did in your everyday life thus showing to people that stopped that they can live without smoking.

The withdrawal symptoms as I mentioned many times is different for each person and are usually mild and are mostly psychological in nature than physical.

When I was writing my first book Thirsty for Health, and I was working on the chapter about Smoking, I wrote that I had terrible withdrawal symptoms. Now after reading Alen Carr's book the Only way to quit smoking I am reevaluating those lines because new elements and information arrived in my mind from that excellent book.

Now I know, and I realized that I didn't have really awful physiological withdrawal symptoms, but they were mostly psychological ones, anxiety, irritation, and alertness are not so many physical signs but mental ones.

I am sure now that my physiological withdrawal symptoms of nicotine were very mild, and I am convinced it was the emotional and psychological aspect that made me believe that I went through severe physical symptoms.

It was like Alan Carrs says in his book 1% physical and 99% psychological ones.

I thought of rewriting the passage about the withdrawal symptoms in Thirsty for health but I will not because it shows how a person's mindset changes when new valid information comes into his way and of course has the open mind to evaluate correctly.

I am quoting the passage, so you see what I mean:

Withdrawals

The three first weeks of stopping to smoke were hell for me. The nicotine withdrawal symptoms started almost immediately after the father, and I had our last cigarette.

I couldn't sleep well—but then again, I hadn't had a restful sleep in years. Stopping smoking wasn't the only reason for my insomnia, but it did intensify it; I could feel a big hole in my chest that was my craving for a cigarette.

I was unfocused, irritable, and I lost my temper very quickly, which is why I didn't get much work done during those days (I didn't want to scare away any customers with my bad mood). I had a constant mental itch in my head as if someone were pricking me with a needle; even today, just thinking about how it felt makes me want to scream.

I also started to eat a lot more than I used to, as my appetite had increased. When I would sit in front of a computer (either installing programs or fixing something hardware- related), I would usually smoke. Now I had to do something else with my hands and my mouth instead so I would eat sandwiches, croissants, chips and drink ice tea and now- caffeinated soda (I gave up caffeine because of my stomach ulcer).

One of the little life experiences that helped me to realize that I could stop smoking and that smoking was not useful or necessary for me was my freedom from caffeine. I figured, "If I could rid myself from caffeine, then why not free myself from nicotine, too?"

I read somewhere that nicotine will leave your body by a fat percentage within three weeks of quitting. I told myself that if I can last for three weeks without smoking, then I will not have any excuse for wanting to smoke because the addictive agent will not be on my system; so that was another reason never to smoke again."

If I drink (alcohol) I will smoke

When I decided to quit smoking back in 2009, I had an advantage in my favor even that at the current period of time I was not aware of it.

I am a very light alcohol drinker for the only reason that I get intoxicated really easy and fast, a gene that I inherited from my mother, I assume she is the same, half a glass of wine and she is off to bed. (smile)

Many smokers that never decide to quit smoking afraid that they will not be able to because in their mindset that's impossible to have a drink and not light a cigarette. This association except having psychological roots also has a profound physiological relationship between alcohol and smoking.

People smoke more tobacco cigs when they drink alcohol because alcohol like stress makes your urine more acidic, the PH of our urine drops dramatically towards the acidic purple end of the spectrum.

Now when a non-smoker drinks alcohol or is under stress, her urine also becomes acidic, but physiologically nothing actually happens to her, in a smoker body thought it's an entirely different story.

When a smoker drinks alcohol or is stressed out, the brain takes the most readily alkaloid substance that finds in the bloodstream and sends it to the urine to make it more alkaline to bring back the correct PH back.

Guess which element? If your answer nicotine, you are correct. The alkaloid effects of nicotine make her the perfect candidate for use from the body.

When that happens, a sudden removal of nicotine from the smoker's bloodstream occurs which equals to an immediate withdrawal symptom which the smoker deals with by lighting a cig to replenish the lost nicotine that went to alkaline her urine.

Like all life in this universe, it's a cycle, in this case, a vicious cycle, you drink alcohol, you create a depletion of your nicotine levels, and then you need to smoke to bring the nicotine levels that your body tolerates back. In a nutshell the more alcohol you drink, the more you smoke.

Actually, if you really made the decision to quit smoking and commit to it then drinking alcohol will expedite the nicotine removal from your body, now I am not telling you to become an alcoholic to stop smoking, but it can work in your favor.

You can quit smoking and drink alcohol at the same time, it's your resolve and commitment that needs to be checked. If you find drinking as an excuse then what's stopping you from using other excuses like I can't drink coffee without a cig, or after eating I must have a cig and so on, do you see the error in this kind of argument?

Learning how to inhale

This is an expression that I was hearing a lot when my smoker friends were remembering when they first started smoking, and they used this phrase, learning how to inhale, and they meant of course how to inhale the smoke of a cig and not the regular good air that contains oxygen.

When people are starting smoking in the beginning when their throat is burning, and they keep going, and they use the phrase learn how to inhale!!! Which is very comic because they only thing that changed was not the ability to find out how to inhale but with regular smoking smokers destroyed the inner lining of nerve cells that are along their windpipe.

These nerve cells are telling you not to inhale smoke down your air pipe because it will lead to death! It's the same cells that prevent you from inhaling smoke and warn you when you are in a fire in a burning building or when you are near a fire like a barbecue or generally encountering smoke.

The next passage is formed my first book Thirsty for Health."

> *After some unfortunate events in my second year in the military, I started tobacco use in a moment of weakness. The irony was that I started smoking the same brand my father had begun smoking when he was in the army—talk about subliminal emotional messages.*
>
> *I was so stupid for starting. I would cough and get dizzy every time I inhaled cigarette smoke, but for some twisted, mindless reason, I would continue to smoke until a cough went away and the*

light-headed feelings were replaced by the addition
of euphoria-inducing nicotine.

Like one of my cousins told me in one of our
many conversations about smoking if the tobacco
industries found a way to make a cigarette that
would have the effect of the smoke and deliver
nicotine to the brain without putting tar in the
lungs, then everybody will smoke. Without knowing
it, my cousin had somehow prophesized the
introduction of electronic cigarettes.

Other Addictions and Smoking.

Society views, beliefs, and opinions on how people with certain addictions should manage to break free or get away from them are not entirely accurate.

As I repeated in this cessation book series and also on my blog, people see smoking as a bad habit and not as a deadly addiction.

For me there are not good habits or bad addictions, there are only bad cravings. There are good habits and bad habits I give you that.

During my studies in Greece except for the smoking addiction I managed to get another addiction namely *StarCraft*. It was a military science fiction computer game which you could choose your race, they were four species, Terrans (humans) The insect-like Zerg's, the very powerful Protos and the very divine Xel'Naga the creator race.

I always played with the Terrans. You could play against the computer, or you could play with another human.

At first, I was playing against the computer, but it took me a short time to figure out the strategy algorithm it was using, and I was winning all the time. The result was that I kind of lost interest. After that and while talking with another friend of mine who also played starcraft he told me that you could play other people, that was it, the phone line was always busy for months after that little information.

My life for about 6 months was revolving around Starcraft games. I was of course addicted. I would eat and drink in front of the computer in case my opponent decides to make a sudden move or a surprise attack. If it weren't for the pause function I would probably move the computer in the toilet, yes that's how addicted I was.

My room was always dark even during the day, I install curtains that blocked sunlight completely, so the only source of light would be my computer monitor, it helped me focus more.

It was when I noticed that people were starting to complain that I miss meeting with them or didn't give them much attention that I realized that hey something is really wrong with me, this thing I was doing this computer game addiction is not exquisite for me.

So what I did was that I just stop playing, the first few days it was so hard when I was sitting in front of the PC to do something else, my hands would automatically try to hit the start craft icon on the screen. My next move was to uninstall the program, and that made things a bit easier, but it took me a while until I stop thinking of playing start craft all the time.

Some will argue that being addicted to a computer game and smoking is not the same, well I disagree, see my 6-month addiction with start craft and the way I managed to break free has a lot in common with quitting smoking and the way I quit smoking.

Stopping playing Starcraft was done cold turkey, that subconsciously let me to the path of using similar tactics with quitting smoking. Uninstalling the program from the computer was like throwing away everything that had anything to do with tobacco use, cigarette packs, lighters, ashtrays, etc.

Some friends of mine gave me attitude after I stopped because they lost a playing partner, the same thing happens with smoking too, people that I used to smoke with complained that I was not their friend anymore and did not hang with them in their deadly smoking sessions!

There are so many other similarities, but you got the picture, what I want to address though is the fact that people that had previous addictions more or less, like Alcoholic Anonymous, use a 12 step method which is, in a nutshell, cold turkey approach. Basically, it tells them to stay away from the substance that makes you have the addiction.

So people that managed to get rid an addiction quitting smoking for them come let's say easier because they realize better, quicker and see the end result more coherent because they have the experience of the past quitting addictions.

For example, people that stop drinking have a better understanding of how to stop smoking because they were satisfied with the way they quit drinking alcohol. They are more aware that even one puff can take them back to full-blown smoking because they know that even a small sip of an alcoholic drink will bring them back to alcoholism!

If I quit smoking, I won't drink (alcohol) again

If you are a light drinker like I am then this should not be an issue. As the days of non-smoking accumulate, you will notice that eating and drinking is more enjoyable than before. The reason is that your senses on a significant physical level start to operate again giving you sensations that smoking deprived of you all those years!

When you reach your second week without smoking as I am sure you will provide you are decided, and you are committed to your quit then you will have a choice for the first time in your life.

You have a choice, you can either continue being a smoke-free person with all the benefits that offers or you can go back to smoking with all the disadvantages it offers.

I am sure that you will choose the smoke-free path and when you do that, you will be faced with smoking triggers. Some of them will be holiday triggers, other will be event triggers and so on. Those triggers many times include alcohol consumption in one way or another. Holidays do tend to be festive, and alcohol flows a bit more than other occasions.

You need to retrain yourself to deal and face them and live them without using the small cylindrical tubes of death between your lips and hands.

So yes if you don't have any alcohol addiction or any other kind of health issues. You can drink your red wine with dinner or have a cold one while watching a game on the telly. You can do everything you did as a smoker as long as you don't have any medical issues or prior addictive behavior.

I smoke whenever and anywhere I want.

Some people are under the illusion that they can continue smoking without taking under consideration societies views and desires and wants and laws!

Twenty and thirty years ago when I was a kid in Cyprus everybody smoked, and they smoked everywhere, it was considered the reasonable thing to do, nobody complained except a few enlightened people who they have been accused by society back then as "troublemakers"!

I know I was there, I could see my father smoke, my uncles smoke, grandfather, elementary and high school teachers, men mostly, women not so much it was considered not ladylike to smoke.

Now thirty years later, and with more people getting informed on smoking's real dangers and the fact that is a drug addiction society is not very tolerated to tobacco use, and that's how it should be.

Now there are laws forbidding smoking in public places, you can't smoke indoors anymore unless you are in your house.

Smoking is banned in the car if you have kids inside and so on. So except the deadly health issues, you will avoid if you quit smoking, you be more socially accepted also.

You just can't go to nonsmoker friends or acquaintances houses and expect to smoke indoors as people did thirty years ago.

I remember people that didn't smoke had ashtrays for their smokers friends to use, it was considered impoliteness if a smoker wanted to smoke and you didn't have an ashtray to offer!!!

Now it completely reverses, and it's a good and correct reverse, now if you go to a house and try to light a cig indoors in a non-smoker room you be yelled at and show you the door. You can smoke outside and not in front of my kids is the usual reply, and I agree with it.

So if you think dear smoker you can smoke where and whenever you want you are sadly mistaken.

If where you live smoking is allowed everywhere, and anywhere then I have news for you, non-smoking is going to catch up to you sooner than you think so what is better quit now or let smoking stop you from your life?

I am not saying this because I am vindictive with smokers, I was a smoker too for sixteen years and is something I regret and will never forget. I am just saying it because that is going to happen and it's a friendly warning that the future doesn't bring any love for smokers. If you are an intelligent person then I am sure you know what to do next, your life, your decision your move. It's better for your health, it's better for your pocket, it's better for everybody around you.

Fifth day Without Smoking.

Physical withdrawal is starting to fade away, and life is starting to become a bit more clear, and your gradual escape from nicotine prison is becoming a reality minute by minute. You realize that you are living your life without smoking is becoming a new lifestyle a new healthy way of life.

You catch yourself feeling new sensations and reevaluating yourself. Fears are still with you, but you have this conviction that you be victorious at the end, because you made the right decision, because you've made a bet with yourself and you are going to win it. You've done a commitment that you will not let anyone or anything, either person situation or a combination of the two to make you smoke again. You are done with smoking,

smoking is for the weak, smoking is for the dump, smoking is simply not for you anymore.

You realized that smoking offered you nothing, absolutely nothing. Smoking is not your friend, your partner, your comfort. Smoking is exactly the opposite of that. Smoking is not your friend, it's your killer, smoking is not your comfort it's your murderer, smoking doesn't offer you anything except black lungs, contrite heart and a life full of disease and illness.

 Only you can retrain yourself to lead a life smoke-free and full of health and happiness, and you are doing a terrific job thus far, and you just need to keep going on.

Every time you wake up in the morning remind yourself why you quit smoking and that only a small puff can ruin your quit and every night before you go to bed thanked yourself for staying smoke-free during the day. In time these morning reminders and night thank you will fade away because smoking will not occupy your head and your heart anymore. You will reach nirvana, you will see smokers, and you will feel sorry for them, pity and empathy for them.

You will notice their mechanical almost robotic movements when they smoke, you will see them as what they really are, drug addicts. With no control what's so ever in their life, and you feel proud of yourself for escaping this prison, you will judge yourself hard for being stupid all those years, and this will reinforce your conviction of never taking another puff in your life.

Sixth Day Without Smoking.

Your sixth day is another day away from the nicotine prison, and it's a signal that you are on your way to a better smoke-free life enriched with the quality of the daily lives moments.

By now you must have noticed changes in your physiology towards the better. Here is a list of the journey you started, and it will show you where are you on the map. It's at the beginning, but like every marvelous and exciting journey, they all start with a small, simple step towards the right direction. You have not trapped anymore into the nicotine illusion and myths. You are an energetic person full of fire ready to embrace life and rediscover yourself. Educate yourself to live without smoking, without heart attacks, without lung cancer without all the dangers of smoking.

Here is a list of what happens after you stop smoking; the effects are phenomenal:

Within 20 Minutes

Your blood pressure returns to its usual level.
Your pulse rate slows to normal.
Your circulation has improved enough that your hands and feet warm to normal body temperature.

Within 4 Hours

Half of the carbon monoxide from your last cigarette has left your bloodstream.

Within 8 Hours

The carbon monoxide from your last cigarette is now gone from your bloodstream. Your blood now carries an average amount of oxygen.

Within 24 Hours

Your chance of a heart attack is lower.

Within 48 Hours

Damaged nerve endings start to re-grow.

Your sense of smell and taste improve.

You are around here right now but don't think about that you have ground to cover. Think and look back of what you achieved thus far. You haven't smoked for six days now, and that's amazing, you should pad yourself on the back and celebrate!

Within 2 Weeks to 3 Months

Your circulation is better.

Walking and physical activity is easier.

Lung function increases up to thirty percent.

Within 1 to 9 Months

You cough less.

You have more energy.

You don't become short of breath as quickly.

The cilia in your lungs re-grow, and you will have less phlegm and infection.

Within 1 Year

Your heart attack risk has fallen to the halfway mark between that of a current smoker and that of someone who has never smoked.

Within 5 Years

If you used to smoke a pack a day, you

have now cut your risk of dying of lung cancer in half.

Your risk of heart attack and stroke approaches that of a non-smoker.

You have cut your risk of mouth, throat, and esophageal cancer by half.

I am here 8 and half years after running. I don't even think about smoking anymore but even that you are there and I am here we both have two things in common, we are both ex-drug addicts in recovery, and it only needs one puff to go back to a full-blown smoker again.

I am sure that you are conviction and your commitment are strong, and you continue to head towards your Freedom from Nicotine.

Within 10 Years

Your chance of dying from lung cancer is almost as small as a non-smoker's.
Your risk of mouth, throat, esophageal, kidney and pancreatic cancer continues to diminish.

Within 10 to 15 Years

Your risk of dying from any cause is almost the same as that of someone who never smoked.

Avoiding situations and places where you used to smoke

This issue is a tricky one. Many people that used the cold turkey method advocate that avoiding as much as possible situations that you used to smoke should be a priority, others advocate that you should not do that because you need to start retraining yourself to live without smoking from day one of your quit.

Both views and opinions are respected, and both stem out from the ex-smokers personal experiences and ordeals.

Personally, I am somewhat in between those two views. I do think that you should stay away from a situation that you used to smoke as much as possible especially the first three days where physiological urges are still in place. After those three days, I agree with the second way of thinking that you should just continue living your life retraining your mind to live without a cigarette and proving to yourself that it's possible and very much doable to have a smoke-free, healthy and happy life.

It's a choice, for example, if when you were a smoker, you used to go out to the porch of your house or your workplace and smoked with other people. Now do not go out when the other people smoke, talk with the non-smokers indoors or wait for the smokers to finish their smoking and speak with them when they come inside.

Another example, when you go to a restaurant to eat, sit in a non-smoking section of the establishment, if your company is smokers then tell them that they can smoke after dinner or they can go to the smoking section of the place, or even outside to smoke. Do not go to the smoking section because your friend or company is a smoker if they are your friends they will indulge and respect your request.

You are going to lose some "friends" in the course of your quit and trust me they were not friends for the first time, you will make new friends believe me and do not despair or think you will stay alone, trust me nobody wants a smelly breathing person for a friend!

Being a non-smoker will make you even more popular with other people because non-smokers are arithmetically more than smokers, you got to love math after that (wink)

Some activities like going to places that they smoke indoors like individual bars or other places you should avoid, second-hand smoke is as bad as firsthand, it doesn't have any nicotine in it, but that doesn't; mean is not still poisonous for you.

You will found new places to spend your time which is smoke-free or provide a non-smoking area, you will make more friends than before, and you will experience new sensations and emotions as your social life is a concern. You will realize that all the years you were under the influence of nicotine you were losing a lot of beautiful and useful items life offers on a daily basis.

My advice after the three days you should attack and tackle every social situation you can get yourself into with an unyielding commitment and conviction that you will go through them without smoking. You need to prove to yourself first and to the people around you that you are serious about quitting tobacco use and it's not just a phase but a fight for your life and the well-being of you and your family.

Closing this section, I want to tell you that associating situations and places and sometimes both with smoking (Nicotine Fix) is not the unique characteristic of the smoker. All addicts of other drugs have the same behavior. They all have places where they take drugs and also the place and time, and the "pleasurable" effect is always controlled by the familiarity of the place.

People usually die from an overdose when they are using their drug (legal or Illegal, doesn't really matter) when they are using in places that never used before.

What I want you to get from this is that for at least the three days avoid situations and places that will trigger a smoking desire in you. If you feel that you need to avoid places for more than three days then, by all means, please do.

Do not though close yourself in 4 walls in your flat or house for longer periods of times like 2 and more weeks. Life goes on, and you need to face reality, you need to re-educate yourself that you can live without the cancer tubes dangling from your mouth.

Smoking and Productivity complete Opposites.

When someone is cold, and he is shaking if you give him or her something to hold he would probably drop it, also if you ask him or her to do anything there is a big chance he would not succeed because he needs to address and solve the shaking issue first before doing anything productive.

When someone is angry or irritated with something he needs first to calm down before he can refocus on what he was doing and start being productive again.

When a smoker doesn't get his nicotine fix on time, which is about every 20 to 30 minutes, it starts to feel and sense early withdrawal symptoms. Irritability, lack of focus, light shaking, headaches a hunger feeling also are some of them, that's why many smokers who smoke for years lost the ability to differentiate the feelings of when they are hungry and when they need to smoke. This leads to overeating because you can only smoke a certain number of cigs before your lungs say enough!

Now all these withdrawal symptoms are all shifting your focus from work to take action either to smoke or to eat.

Now this means you need to stop what you are doing to satisfy the urge and this often happens when you are a smoker.

A smoker averages every hour, if he can leave his post at work, smokes 2 times that's about 10 to 15 minutes average away from his work and thus not working. In an 8-hour work schedule, a smoker works less from 1hour and 20 minutes to 2 hours!

Apparently, employees that smoke is less productive than their non-smoker colleagues.

Also, add the time that smokers leave their workplace to eat, take a private phone call or use the toilet.

What smokers afraid is non-existent, if they quit smoking they will become more productive because the time wasted to satisfy their addiction can be spent on working! What smokers afraid is not real, they associated the ability on focusing on work with smoking which has nothing to do with each other.

They associate the potential to focus on their task with smoking, like all the other events in their life. They wake up, and they think that lighting a cigarette will help them get out of bed, they drink their coffee, and they believe that by smoking they will make the coffee drinking more enjoyable. They talk on the phone, and they smoke at the same time thinking it will help them listen better, it's all hocus pocus and psychological fears that were created with years of smoking. The only thing smoking does is not assist you in focus or be more productive or wake up or enjoy other aspects of your daily life, the only thing that smoking does is to deliver a highly noxious addictive substance into your brain and bloodstream enslaving your soul deeper with every puff to the nicotine prison.

I am sure that by now you caught yourself finding more time to do things. You need to see this accumulative. When I was smoking 40 cigs a day, I was "lucky" because back then in Greece the no indoor smoking law was not in effect yet. After when I came back to Cyprus, and I was working as a college professor, I couldn't smoke inside I had to go out to smoke and that's when I started feeling like an outcast. That's when I started looking the pitiful looks other people were giving me from a distance and also when I was talking to them I now remember that they kept their distance apparently because of my breath sticking smoke.

But now you don't have that smelly issue your breath is amazing and fresh, and you don't have that problem anymore.

Anyway back to my point, instead of correcting papers and grading papers on my off time or reading something relevant to my work or socializing with other people I would go outside and smoke, killing myself and alienating myself from other people and only hanging out with other pitiful smokers. Also, I think of all that time I lost by smoking, and I realize how much more I could do for me or for my work at the college.

That's why since I stop smoking and especially the last years bringing my weight down to normal after briefly flirting with obesity I make sure every second of my life from now own to be spent in a useful manner first for me and secondly for the people around me.

You need to be a little selfish, you need to have a little ego that will make you see that you should do things for you once, make that a number one priority stop try to satisfy everyone else first and then yourself. Being a little selfish is a healthy attitude.

Quitting smoking would be for you and nobody else, your precious health and your precious life should be motive enough to make the decision to commit yourself to stop smoking.

You are on an excellent road and in a safe place now, you were on the bottom of the pit, and you can only go up from now, life will only get better from now on. Stick to your commitment, and you will see that the smoke-free version of you is cable off so much more, things that you never thought possible.

I mean when I quit smoking I never thought that 2 years after that I would finish my first marathon! I never dream that I would be able to run 42km and 195 meters.

Your smoke-free future is going to be heaven!

Why would anyone go back to smoking?

Since 2009 I am tobacco free, and I now know that smoking is stupid. Does that mean that for the 16 years I was a smoker I was also stupid as well? The answer to that question I am afraid is yes, for sixteen years I was an idiot, dumb, stupid and most important of all I was swimming in "blissful" ignorance.

People that smoke is in their majority intelligent people, smart but somehow they act like their IQ is lower than a potato and potatoes IQ is not even zero is non-existent!!!

What makes clever people behave so stupidly? I tell you what? Nicotine addiction, a smoker doesn't choose to smoke, he is a prisoner of the addictive powers of nicotine.

When I started learning about nicotine, and the information began to saturate my thick ignorance head that I started waking up and on a conscious level began to see what I am doing to myself.

My thoughts were cloudy for the most of my life, for 16 years and I know now that smoking was the reason.

Why on earth would someone want to go back to smoking? I am sure you will never go back to smoking because you see smoking of what it is, a useless addiction that you are successfully getting rid off and escaping the nicotine trap and prison.

I can only see two reasons for someone to go back to smoking. One if she or he wants to die prematurely and have a degraded quality of life then sure smoking is perfect for them. The second reason is if you really enjoy the withdrawal symptoms of quitting mostly psychological one then you should smoke a cigarette every three days because that's how many days it needs for the bulk of the nicotine to get out of your system. If you really like the withdrawal symptoms yes go back to smoking!

Do not let psychological triggers trick you into starting smoking again, be smarter than the addiction not stronger, take the battle to a place that you will have the most chances of winning.

Your intellect is your ally, not your emotional state is going t help you if an urge comes, I am repeating that the urges are mostly psychological by now, use your brain, do not let anything else make the decision.

Decide not to smoke, and you be fine, the urge will go away very soon, and you can continue with your life a happy camper.

Triggers that urge you to Smoke.

I remember when I was university student I would go and watch movies on cinema almost every week and I remember distinctly that a few minutes before the film starts there was a barrage of commercials mostly sodas and always Coca-Cola. I didn't think about it much back then, but now I know that one of the reasons I will always drink coca cola and watch a movie is because subconsciously I associate and this is the key word, associated watching movies and drinking Coke.

I mean before I go into the viewing room of the cinema they were a range of other liquid products I could buy from the shops outside, but I always got Coke without thinking, why is that? Well from a big part it was the commercial that made me associate that I cannot have the one without the other.

I remember that once I went to a movie theater that only serves Pepsi not Coke and me became really irritated for no reason, I mean it's a beverage for goodness sake. I didn't enjoy the movie that day even if the movie kick ass as quality was concerned because they didn't have coke so I could drink while watching the film.

Now this irritation was not physical, I didn't get a physiological withdrawal symptom because I didn't have Coke to drink it was only in my head.

Now I stopped drinking Coke long before I quit smoking and for some years every time I was going to the cinema or watched a movie. I could feel this urge to get a Coke, but every time I would say to myself that I was done with Coke. It's not healthy for me, and I restrained myself not to want Coke anymore.

Same trigger principle is going to apply with your smoking triggers. If you were like me a heavy smoker, where the only time at some point in my life I didn't smoke was when I was asleep you are going to have more smoking triggers than the smoker that only smokes 2 to 5 cigs.

My smoking triggers that I had were, while fixing computers, back then I had a small computer shop, I would sell and repair computers. So when I was setting them or installing software, I would always smoke.

Another smoking trigger was after food, I stopped drinking coffee a few years before, so I didn't have the coffee trigger with me when I stop smoking, so I guess that was a blessing. Something less to worry about.

There were the major smoking triggers that were of personal nature then I had the more social related smoking triggers like having a beer or alcohol with friends on a night out I would want to smoke, or going to parties and other people will smoke.

Or family gatherings on holidays or other events where all my cousins and uncles were also smoking.

The important thing about a smoking trigger is to recognize and accept that you want a cigarette but chose not to have one because you know now that the tradeoff is much better for you now. Your motive is the realization that your health is the most important thing in your life.

I don't remember where I told this story before, but I think there is a perfect time to mention it again.

When I was in high school one of my favorite professors gave us an example, the funny thing was that he used a mathematical representation and he was an Ancient Greek professor.

He told us that health is number 1 and he wrote on the blackboard using his white choke the number 1.

Then he said let's say your parents gave you 10 dollars and he wrote a zero next to the 1 making it a ten. Then he said let's say your godmother gave you 100 dollars for your birthday and he wrote another zero next to ten making it 100 and we continue doing that until the number on the board was 1 000 000 dollars!

Then he said now you are a millionaire but without your health and with a theatrical sword like move deleted number one from the board. Without your health, you are nothing showing the six zeros that left on the board.

That was an image that stuck with me for a long time until I smoke my first cig! Of course, this small story from my teacher really helped me after to evaluate and understand how important my health is.

Every person is unique do not compare your quit with other people quits.

When I was a student at the university, I had a terrible habit which was paying too much attention to what other people were doing concerning their studies instead of focusing on mine. I was comparing my results I had with other people's result, and from that comparison, I was justifying possible failures I had.

For example, if I got a 3 out of 10 and saw that the rest of the students on average they got a 5 out of 10 then I will justify my failure by saying see even the kids that study really hard only got 5 so my 3 its ok I actually went well on this exam!!!

This kind of rationalizations to justify and conceal my failure were a big part of my life until at some point I realized that all my fellow students finished their studies and I was still there rationalizing my failures and in the process staying put!

A 5 out of 10 is a passing point, and you don't have to take that exam again, my 3 was not that was the difference. My fellow friends and students were going forward with their studies I, on the other hand, was not because my mind instead of working to help me I was wasting time on useless comparisons.

A similar tactic occurs with smokers too and also with smokers who compare their quit with other quits of other people.

They will start a quit last a week and then light a cig, and they rationalize their failure by saying well at least I lasted a week George or Steve, or Ann only lasted three days, like it's a contest of something!!!

Or the first three days they will be talking on the phone with an ex-smoker and the ex-smoker will tell them I didn't have any significant withdrawal symptoms. You, on the other hand, are having some severe nicotine withdrawal symptoms and you are thinking maybe something is wrong with you or you are not doing something right or-or-or.

Another thing smokers do is to compare their own previous quits with the current one, saying stuff like last time I didn't feel that bad during the first three days, or these time I catch myself eating a lot more and many similar comparisons.

Every quit is unique even your own previous quits have nothing to do with each other because if you think about it, you are not the same person you were the last time you tried to quit. Every second that passes we acquired new information's, new experiences and our brain is reshaping itself to understand and utilize this new information, in reality at the cellular level we are a different person from second to second!

Comparing your quit with other people or with your own previous ones will not help you at all, and it will jeopardize your success.

Focus on your current quit, take it day by day, when you have urges acknowledge them and then chose not to smoke, you are in charge of your life not a substance like Nicotine, be smarter than Nicotine not stronger, you can do it.

Long-Term Ex-Smokers who say they have "Bad Days."

Refers to people that after they quit smoking, they might have thoughts of tobacco use and they are describing that day as a rough day. This kind of behavior might make people think that it will always be like that in the future forever if they quit. The truth of the matter is not at all like that. As you get more time under your belt as an ex-smoker and as you educate and train yourself to deal with new triggers effectively, this kind of urges will go away. At some point you will reach a level, in which I am now, that you will not believe you were a smoker ever, you will forget that you smoked and that's an amazing feeling to have to reach that level of clearing all the associations of smoking from your thoughts and from your life.

You will reach a level where tobacco will be so disgusting to you that you will make sure people that smoke closes the doors and windows so the smoke will not get back inside the room you are either at work or home.

When you see people smoke you will feel sorry for them, and you will keep your distance, so you don't get that second-hand smoke in your face.

You be able to notice the drug addict almost robotic movements a smoker does, light a cig, takes a puff then exhales, take a puff again until the cig is finished and then most probably if there is no ashtray around he or she will throw the filter bud on the ground!

205

There are no bad days in the future because an ex-smoker thinks he wants a cig, even if he wants one, it was probably a trigger an event that happened a long time ago and didn't have the chance to cope with it without smoking. As a result, his brain will create those new neuron patterns that will educate you that hey you can do this without smoking you can go through this event smoke-free.

People like to present something they accomplished as being really hard, it gives them a sense of accomplishment, I fell into that trap too when I was writing my first book Thirsty for Health I said that I had terrible withdrawal symptoms. Now that I am reviewing the information I read and also doing some memory exercises and remembering my quitting period, I didn't have terrible withdrawal symptoms, it was mostly psychological symptoms I didn't shake like a leave every time I had the urge to smoke.

I remember I felt irritated a lot, I remember being uneasy, couldn't focus very well the first few days. I had a feeling I was hungry all the time, and that is how nicotine withdrawal feels like, but it was not the symptoms that classical mythology on smoking describes that its difficult to quit smoking because of terrible withdrawal symptoms.

It's 99% psychological and 1% physiological once you grasp that you are going to be free from the nicotine trap really fast and easy, as I am sure you are doing right now being on your sixth day and continuing strong smoke-free and becoming healthier by the minute.

Chapter 6
Second Week Of Your Freedom

Your first Monday morning as a non-smoker

When I write in my blog (thirsty4health.com) and also in my books about running and also weight loss, I always encourage people to keep a diary to catalog their activities.

There are a lot of reasons why you should do that, and they are all beneficial. When you feel sick or under the weather you can always check out your diary, see what you ate and drunk what kind of exercise you did what the climatic conditions were and you can make some really useful concluded results about what causing you to be sad or sick or happy et cetera.

When for years smokers abuse their body they go through a particular range of illnesses and patterns, their body does its best to get rid of the nicotine off, and that's why you are able to smoke in the first place. If the liver didn't remove the nicotine from our body, we would be dead in a matter of hours after smoking about 20 cigarettes, that's how toxic nicotine is, just imagine that is used as the primary ingredient in pesticides! And is responsible in significant part for the death of the bees around the globe.

Back to my point, smokers think that smoking doesn't do anything to their health that's how much the nicotine fried their brains, if you ask a smoker why he has pneumonia he will say because of a bug or because of the cold weather it's never the smoking!!! That's how ignorant, and under the addiction smokers are, don't get me wrong I know exactly how they feel. I was a pathetic, pitiful smoker not so long ago, I actually believed that smoking was just a bad habit nothing to do with my health as colds or flues or other minor health issues were concerned! I actually remember arguing and talking with other smokers saying that it was never proven that smoking causes lung cancer! Ignorance is not bliss, it kills.

What about cancer? Someone will say well the mind of smoker is that cancer is for other people, it will not happen to me! Typical drug addict rationalization, no logical at all, rationalized enough just to allow the brain to give the permission to continue smoking!

After the smoker stops to smoke the body starts to work overtime. Because now the bulk of nicotine is out of your system it only has to deal with toxins of the tar. This way it becomes more efficient at cleaning all the bad stuff.

When this process happens and especially the first few months, the smoker might experience a range of physiological and psychological changes and also events, some of them are bad and have a dose of discomfort and other most of them are very beneficial and healthy for you.

So on your sixth day, you might feel fantastic, or you might feel crappy and generally not in the mood, what you need to remember is that you be feeling the same way even if you smoke. Do not blame your quit for the bad psychological state you are in or your physiological situation on the fact that you quit smoking.

People that are in their quit process (I am talking with Cold Turkey Method always) tend to blame any new non-beneficial change in their life to quit smoking, but when it is a beneficial change like the food taste better, you don't see them padding their back for quitting smoking. They remember that they quit tobacco use and blame that as their cause of bad karma when something uncomfortable happens(like the flu or constant coughing) The truth is that quitting smoking is the best thing that happened to you and what you feel, or sense will happen either you smoke or not.

What drives people that are on their quit and particular the first days to think like that is they didn't manage and didn't learn yet how to get rid off completely the association of living and smoking. This is going to be a work in process, and at some point, you will break the union that you need a cigarette to live or continue your life or deal with life events. Trust me on this, you will reach a point where you will see other people smoke and feelings of pity and compassion towards the poor addict will emerge.

If you quit last Tuesday, then Monday would be your sixth day without cigs, and you might complain that you had an atrocious Monday. Like you had difficulty waking up in the morning, and you had a bad day at work you had to do things you didn't like, and you somehow blame the fact that you don't smoke anymore. You are demonizing the lack of smoking of being responsible for all the things you didn't like or did not pan out the way you were hoping.

In reality, the things you didn't like were happening when you were a smoker, hating to wake up in the morning or a mishap happening at work are things that have nothing to do with smoking or not smoking. It's the chronic psychological association that makes you think it has.

Other people will say that their weekend was so beautiful and smooth and relaxing and they didn't have so much urges to smoke but coming Monday they started having these feelings of anxiety and stress. They had to face for the first time in a long time a Monday without tobacco use, and that made them assume that not smoking is responsible for their Monday events which are entirely false and utterly illogical.

Second Week without Smoking

If you followed the advice that I gave in the first book series that you should start your quit on a Tuesday then your second week without smoking begins on a Monday. Your first Monday without smoking! You might find it difficult to wake up or blame everything that went wrong at the house or at work because of quitting smoking. The truth is that you stopping tobacco use and having a bad day has nothing to do with each other, you were going to have a bad day anyway smoking or not smoking. I might repeat myself here, but I think it's important to understand this issue I am pointing out, which is having a bad day doesn't have to do anything with you quitting smoking. The events are completely un-associated with each other.

When I stopped smoking, I don't think it was a Tuesday, but I am sure it was a work day it was definitely not a weekend. I wish I knew the things I am telling you in this book back then, my quit would have been easier on me as my mental status concern.

If I stopped a Tuesday, then I would have gone through my regular routine for three working days Tuesday, Wednesday, and Friday without smoking and I would have educated myself, proved to myself that I can live without a cigarette, improving my self-esteem at the same time and also my self-confidence.

Also, I would have gone through the motions and the social interactions of a weekend, my first weekend without smoking, repeating the same basic action of identifying an urge, acknowledging and choosing not to smoke.

On a cellular level nicotine is stronger than us, that's why we smoke in the first place anyway, we are addicted to it, but on an intellectual level, we are definitely smarter than nicotine!

So bring the fight to your own ground, where all the advantages and the odds are for you.

Acknowledge the urge and then do the smart thing, do not smoke and continue doing what you were doing before the call came.

This is the right and an easy and only way to quit smoking not as I did it, it was cold turkey, and I am 100% behind this method. It is the only one that has the most successful quits but the psychological aspect and the way I went to stop smoking it was wrong. I used my will to quit, I was one of the lucky ones I guess, but now I see that there is a much easier way and it's the way I just described in a nutshell just now.

Now you are on Monday your first Monday without smoking, and you know you are ok because you have a week of not smoking under your belt, you faced most of your working triggers and also most of your weekend triggers. I am sure your self-confidence is up and is continuing to get up with every day that passes without smoking. You prove to yourself that you own this you can do this, you are in charge now of your life, you have two weeks of experience under your belt, you are not green anymore.

This week is going to be much much easier because your new found experiences are going to help you overcome it, you are not starting your quit now you are well 7 days into your quit and going strong with it. Your self-esteem is also up and will continue to go up with every urge you manage successfully to postpone and kick away.

You will see that by the end of this week you will not have so many urges as before and also the urges that you may have are purely psychological and have nothing to do with the addictive nature of nicotine, the nicotine has left your body, Elvis has left the building people(smile).

Now you will not have any excuse to smoke, nicotine is out, the addictive agent is no longer in your body.

Now it's a matter of retraining and relearning to live without smoking in your life.

After I quit smoking, I have lots of Headaches

I was a smoker for 16 years, and I remember I was buying and using a lot of paracetamol, or panadol and aspirin and other painkillers and pain reliever drugs

I now know that a significant contributor and sometimes the culprit of my headaches and especially lots of migraines was the fact that I was a smoker. How do I know that? Well, first indicator was that after I had stopped smoking those awful headaches stop happening, which was a blessing in two ways, first that meant I stop inflicting to my body pain through smoking and second I started saving money on painkillers and aspirin.

Don't kid or fool yourself, one in two smokers dies because of tobacco use and the rest a fat percentage ends up as a cripple for life with illnesses like emphysema. *Smoking kills* a slogan that people end up not taking seriously anymore. Maybe a new slogan should be issued like Nicotine kills which are is more direct and address the problem to its core.

Saying that there are other reasons that people have headaches and smoking maybe doesn't have a role to play in it. The only way to see if smoking causes your headaches is to stop tobacco use and determine whether they end if they stop then you can say with pretty much certainty that hey smoking was the cause of my misery and the fact that I had to take painkillers 5 to 6 times a day! That's what happened with me. Now if you stop smoking and still have headaches then you should check it out with a doctor see what the cause is.

The Economic aspect of the nicotine addiction.

How much money I spent on cigarettes, I think if I took all that money and burned them instead of buying cigs it would have kept me warm for a lot of cold nights during the winter season!

I remembered years ago it must have been in 2002 when I was visiting my girlfriend in England and cigs were so expensive that I was buying the cheap ones and in the back of my mind, I was thinking wow I got a good deal! Not even registering that I was killing myself.

See my mindset back then was that cigarettes were a product, which it is for the tobacco company, but for me, it was a product that I thought I needed, that it was necessary for me, that was useful for me.

Not even the cost of cigarettes made me realize that hey you crazy drug addict wake up, it took me years to end up being in a situation where I was scared for my life and for my quality of life. It was then that I realized that the tradeoff of quitting smoking for my health and my life was worth it.

Let me ask you this? If you quit smoking, I give you a million dollars how that made you feel on a psychological level? I am sure your commitment to stop would be through the roof because of the trade-off, quitting smoking for one million dollars in an addicts mind is worth it, then why can't you have the same commitment and attitude towards your health primarily and the health of your family secondary?

Why do we consider our health as something granted and most dangerous of all we feel that our health will never be in danger!

The hard truth is that cigarettes are not a product that you need, it's not a product that is useful, it's a poison that removes your will to lead your life as you would like to live and you let nicotine life your life as she wants.

If you want to go to the movie theatre from 8 p.m. to 10 p.m. to watch a movie, then you should be able to do that without needing to go out every 30 minutes to smoke.

You should be able to enjoy your coffee as it really is, taste the majestic flavor and smell the wonderful aroma of the coffee. With smoking, you can't really enjoy that because your sense of smell and taste are destroyed and compromised from that 4000 chemicals the tobacco plant has, and they are messing with your body.

I did smoke less thought while I was in England because I couldn't afford to buy the volume of cigarettes I was doing when I was in Greece where cigs were much much cheaper.

So in a sense, I did smoke less, but that did not urge me to quit, so the policy of the government to increase the price on cigs doesn't actually help people quit smoking, on the contrary, the smoker will find other ways to get cheaper cigs

I have an idea which I think it will work if the governments of this planet really want to make their citizens quit smoking, then they should pass a law that says all cigarette packets should be sold 1 cent of the dollar only.

Cigarettes should be that cheap, 1 cent for 20 cigs a pack. The government should remain in force this law, smokers will love it, I mean 1 cent per 20 cigarettes wow I can smoke as much as I want and not worry about money.

If the governments of this planet make sure that cigs are sold to their countries with that price tobacco companies will stop producing cigs because they will stop making money, they will probably start making another kind of products that are not so harmful for human consumption.

After you quit, you will find something to improve yourself.

When I quit smoking in 2009, from 2009 until 2010, I was basically retraining myself to live without tobacco use, and I pretty much work myself a lot, I became a workaholic from a shopaholic (smile), and I sadly replaced food with smoking.

But stopping smoking was one of the pivotal moments in my life because it sparked a beginning that brought me to my current situation which I am so grateful.

216

After stopping smoking, I gained a lot of weight, and with the already accumulated weight, I was flirting with obesity.

So I started running to lose the weight, and after reaching a level of where I wasn't losing any more weight, I discover the lifestyle or whole plant-based diet which basically opens the door to the amazingly healthy and happy life I am living right now.

After quitting smoking, I felt that an enormous weight had lifted from my chest and I think it has merit both on the physiological aspect and also with my psychological situation.

I found out and it was a pleasant surprise that now I could sleep better, I was getting rested more easily I didn't have to stop what I was doing because I needed to smoke. The time I was wasting smoking I was using now to do other things more productive especially for my work and also for my personal time.

Also the end of the month I had more money in my bank account, and sure it was nice, I could use that money for me, for my family and anything else I think it's worth spending them on.

By stopping smoking I personally rediscover running, and in the course, I fell in love with it again, and it became a lifestyle for me which is with me until today.

Running makes me feel amazing, it helps with my health and also keep me fit, I feel 15 years younger every time I run, and it is a huge positive improvement in my life.

Another significant improvement in my life and it's indirectly caused by the fact that I stopped smoking is the fact that for the last two years I am writing and self-publishing books which have a huge beneficial positive effect on my life and most importantly on my psyche.

I know many people that after they had quit smoking, they grab the opportunity to do something with the extra time and extra money they found themselves having by developing individual skills or acquiring new hobbies some of them even went back to college or started doing a master or a Ph.D. in their favorite subjects.

In a nutshell, quitting smoking except having an immediate impact on your health it opens numerous opportunities to do something else with your life and is always most of the time beneficial for your quality of your life and for the lives of the people that consist your inner and outer social circle.

I want to smoke one cigarette.

When I quit smoking back in 2009 using the Cold Turkey Method, I didn't do it right. Hopefully, you are doing it the correct way. Now you are into your second week without the tubes of death in your life. My mistake back then was that I quit smoking using the method of willpower, I am not saying people can't stop like that, I mean I did it like that but it has some nasty surprises along the way into the future.

When someone is stopping with willpower, it cannot understand the physiological and psychological symptoms, and as a result, he or she cannot separate which urge to smoke is physiological and which is psychological.

Trying to be stronger than nicotine (willpower) is a bad idea. It's a bad idea because you will stay smoke-free until a trigger in the

218

future so powerful will come along that will challenge your willpower, and your chances of losing to nicotine again are high.

The right mental and psychological state of mind that someone wants to quit is first to admit that he is a drug addict and second to take the high roll and realize that you must be smarter than nicotine not stronger.

When the urge to smoke came instead of taking a very useful pause and identify it as a nicotine wanting, I would panic, and I would do actions that would occupy my mind until the urge would go away.

Doing that yes I was allowing myself to clean its self from nicotine, but I was not educating myself mentally of why I was doing it. Trust me when I say this, quitting smoking is probably 1% physical symptoms (nicotine) mostly the first 3 days and 99% psychological associations that you need to break and retrain yourself to live without a cigarette.

What I should have done was whenever an urge was coming to take a valuable pause, and if I was in the first three days then acknowledge the fact that I want a cigarette and then define why I want one. I wanted one because my nicotine levels dropped and I needed to replenish them. After doing that I CHOOSE not to smoke and I could accomplish that by doing some tips that I already mentioned in the book like brushing my teeth with mint toothpaste, or chewing a sugarless chewing gum or take deep breaths, etc.

Now if I had an urge to smoke let's say the 8th day of my quit where nicotine is not that of an issue any more then I would pause and acknowledge the fact that I want to smoke and then recognize that the urge is of psychological nature. This way I can be more easily choose not to smoke because I know that it's not a real urge is in my head, and I can do something else until the thought leaves my mind. I could go for a walk, walking always clears our head from overloading and overbearing negative thoughts. I could have called my brother or my sister or a friend to talk with them until the urge goes.

This is the smarter way to quit smoking, be more intelligent than nicotine not stronger (willpower) than nicotine.

Future triggers of you wanting to smoke will emerge, I mean I smoke-free since 2009 now, and I might have 2 urges a year to smoke, but now I know that are psychological urges and only last like a split of a second. Now I apply the smarter approach than the willpower path. I am aware that I will not smoke again for the rest of my life because I know I am a drug addict in recovery for life and it only needs one puff to go back being a sick, pitiful stupid smoker!

I value my life too much now and also living tobacco-free for so many years now it's the best proof that the way I am now, it's much much better from a smoker's life.

I am convinced you are smoke-free well into your second week, being smarter than nicotine and starting to see what a wonderful life is without smoking.

Dreaming of Smoking

The first days of quit smoking I was a little bit edgy, but I now know that the physical withdrawal was not that bad it was more the psychological aspect of my status quo that caused me to be on the edge of the razor. Then I was not in a position to recognize what I was having and why I was having the symptoms I had. If I knew the information I now know then I would be able to acknowledge that it was the feeling of fear of

220

the unknown, what do I do after quit smoking? Also, a lot of myths I thought they were the truth was not making my psyche rest and deal with calmness and intelligence my situation.

I do remember though that I started sleeping better, but the funny thing is that I didn't have any dreams. We always dream every night, of course, that's one of the many ways of the brains optimization options to keep itself in good working order. I was just not remembering my dreams.

So at the early stages of my quit, I did not have any dreams revolving around smoking.

Quite recently I remembered a dream which scared the living sh*t out of me. The dream was so intense and realistic I actually woke up thinking that I threw my quit away.

I dreamed that I smoke a cigarette and the soonest I took a few puffs I got so scared that I woke up. I jumped out of bed and walked around the house for a few minutes to shake off the dream. Until I got my bearings right I was so scared because I thought that I actually smoked a cigarette, the only thing I didn't do was to start searching for the filter! What made the whole thing more surreal was that I could actually taste and smell the cigarette I smoked in my dream! But how was that possible? There was no smoke.

I was lucky because that the time I saw that dream was the time period I was researching about this book and I found out it turns out a lot of ex-smokers have them as well and actually will have them in the future.

The reason I had that smoking dream is that after I stopped smoking my cilia the natural brooms that are in your lungs start to function again and they start removing all that tar from the lungs.

What happened was while I was dreaming the tar from my lungs came up and picked up by my taste buds and nose. Luck has it at the same time I was dreaming about smoking, and that made the whole scenario more intense and realistic.

After researching online and especially checking one of Joel Spitzer videos about this matter(link the video here, you should treat the ebooks like a huge article.), it turns out the fact that I woke up scared and panicked is a good thing. It's a good thing because I woke up from a nightmare and not a dream and because I was so afraid that I lost my quit means I am on the right track of viewing smoking as it really is a dangerous addiction.

Many people might say that because you dream of smoking it means that you have to start smoking again, no that's not the case at all it only means that you still have tar in your lungs and sometimes your senses pick them up and create this weird matrix effect on you.

Now I know, and now you know that if I dream or your dream in the future about smoking again is a good thing because it means my lungs and your lings are getting rid of of all the bad stuff that was accumulated all the years that I smoked.

Getting sick after quitting smoking

When I was a smoker I used to get colds, flu and sometimes pneumonia and I didn't get well soon, it would take a week to ten days sometimes just to feel better. Now if I were wiser and not a stupid drug addict I would have interpreted that as a severe warning and would have changed the way I live and behave, but when you are young and restless well you are just that, young and dumb!

After I had quit smoking, of course, I got colds and the flu, but that was not because I quit smoking it was because my immune system was down and the bugs and virus found fertile ground to do what they do best to multiply!

Do not blame quitting smoking for colds you get after, on the contrary, because you quit smoking gradually and with combination with exercise and proper nutrition your immune system will get better, and you will get fewer colds and flu, and when you get them it won't last for days.

Since I stop smoking, I don't remember my colds or my flu's to last more than 2 days! And on another note, since I adopted running and whole plant-based diet as a lifestyle I don't remember getting the flu at all!

In a nutshell, see you quitting smoking as a blessing for your health and for your quality of life. Quitting smoking will allow you to have fewer illnesses and diseases and enable you to experience a more active tobacco-free life.

People smoking in front of you

The first week of my quit I made sure not to be in social contact with people that smoke because in the back of my mind looking other people smoke while I was on my quit process it was too much for me to handle. I made a decision that at least for the first week I will avoid most social events that have to smoke as their central theme. Like going out for a coffee even that I stop drinking coffee I went out with friends that drink coffee and smoke, I would have tea and smoke, or soda, usually ice tea.

When I went into my second week though I had to go out in the world, I had a computer shop running at the time, and it would not operate by itself.

The difference of the second week thought was that the urges were not as often and intense (intensity for every person is different and unique) and my self-esteem and self-confident were boosted. For the first time in my life, I was sure in my bones that I own this, that this quit would be the last one, that I was going to be able to set free from the deadly trap and prison of nicotine.

With time watching other people smoking was less of an issue for me, and at the point I am now every time I watch people smoke feelings of sympathy, empathy and pity surge up my psyche. I just can't stop thinking that not so many years ago I was in their shoes, killing myself from the inside out, destroying my health, ruining my social circle, throwing away my hard earned money.

Living and Getting on with the rest of your Life.

By now you are free from Nicotine, that toxic substance is not flowing through your veins anymore, and it's not saturating your brains receptors, simply is not there, you are for the first time in your life free from it, and you should be really proud of your accomplishment.

As long as you stay away from all possible and alternative ways of putting into your body nicotine you be a happy and healthy camper.

The secret now is this, for the first time you have a choice, you can either go back to smoking or not too is that simple. Now that you are free and for the first time in your life, you can make the decision for yourself without being under the hypnotic state of a bloody sick promoting addictive drug like nicotine is.

I am 100% sure that you will choose the tobacco (nicotine)-free option, is better for your health, is better for your pocket it's better for the people around you.

Will you encounter triggers that will make you want a cigarette? Of course, you will, but from my experience, smoking will not be in your mind anymore.

The one thing you must always be alert and deal with it is the fact that all the future urges you will have or dreams about smoking you will have are all in your mind. The desires to smoke at this particular time are an illusion created by the years of associate everything you did with tobacco use and embedding tobacco use in your life as it's your friend.

If you remember this then you be ok and nothing to worry about.

By now you faced and came victorious with your most common daily smoking triggers now slowly but gradually you be called upon to meet all the other events of your life that for many years you used to go through with smoking.

From my experience when one year passed I had this very fulfilling feeling and content that I was going to make it that I was free at last from the psychological grab of smoking which is much much stronger than the real pull of nicotine.

For you it might be sooner or later than my one year, nobody knows, and you are the only one that will find out.

For me it took about a year to encounter all my smoking triggers and face them others might need more or less.

You will have name day triggers, and birthday triggers of your own or your friends, you will have summer smoking triggers, and winter smoking triggers, especially winter ones that you are closed into your house and sometimes boredom sets in, you should be prepared for this kind of situations.

Christmas holidays and New Years Eve holidays, Easter and Halloween If you are an American or any other religious or not position that you used to smoke now you have to keep a clear mind, be smarter than nicotine and choose not to smoke.

Try to reduce your caffeine and alcohol intake they are not right for yourself, now if you are drinking a glass of wine now and then or have a cup of Jo rarely when you go out with friends that are not a big deal. Unless you suffer from caffeinism and you are alcoholic, then I strongly suggest you stay away from coffee and alcohol.

Keep applying the day by day algorithm, do not think about the future and what it will be without smoking.

Wake up in the morning and commit to yourself that you will not smoke today like you have been doing for the last two weeks, then face the urges when they arrive, do not bother your mind with if's if it comes. When the urge comes, you will know it's an illusion it's not real, acknowledge it and then choose not to smoke. There are many ways to kill an urge, and I already mentioned them here, but the most efficient and the one you can use anywhere and everywhere is taking deep breaths until the urge goes away.

After it goes away repeat this to yourself, *I sure love not smoking* and pad yourself on the back.

When night finally sets in, and you go to bed pad yourself on the back again and congratulate your beautiful self for making through another day without smoking.

Sometimes we need to remind ourselves.

What keeps people from escaping smoking is the physical withdrawal, and by now you are over it, and if you sit down and think about that statement, it wasn't that hard after all. I know that you might disagree with me if you had harsh nicotine withdrawal symptoms but if you actually close your eyes and think back then when you had you irritation or your lack of focus that the physical symptoms were not that hard.

When I stopped smoking in 2009, I thought that I went through hell with the withdrawal symptoms and I wrote that to my first book as well, Thirsty for health. The reality of the matter was that yes I had physical withdrawal symptoms, but they were not the hell I thought I went through. The thing that I know now that was really bothering back them was that I was so frustrated and irritated because I didn't know how long this situation will last. Which is top 3 days and basically I was in ignorance and if I knew the facts that I described in my previous books and also this book I would have had a better withdrawal status.

It is a good practice to stay away from friends and relatives that smoke on these early days, and attack those situations later when your confidence is better.

It is a good idea to make friends that are not smokers, and this will act as reinforcement as for why you quit. Being around people that do not smoke, is healthy for you and you can see first hand that hey, you can live without having a cigarette in your hand and mouth every 30 minutes. You are able to embrace and acknowledge the fact that for the first time for many years now

227

you are free for real and that the smoke of addiction is not clouding your judgment anymore.

Why will anyone go back to smoking?

Right now you know how careless smoking is, and probably hate yourself for being so dumb for so many years, I had and still have the same thoughts until today. The stupidity of the matter is so big that sometimes I hit myself on the head for allowing a drug control and destroy my life and my health for so many years, sixteen years was my "magic" number, unfortunately.

But do not despair, 24 hours after you quit you already added 5 years to your lifespan. Isn't that amazing? We are so lucky to have an amazing body as the human body is.

We are so preoccupied of poisoned this fantastic, magnificent piece of God's engineering that because of its resilience we take it for granted, we don't think that we only have one heart and if she breaks then sayonara baby, nest scene is you in a coffin 6 feet under!

You are on the right track, you escaped that physical withdrawal, the nicotine is not in your system anymore, you have no physiological reason to smoke, the excuse that I am addicted and I must smoke is not valid for you now, nicotine is out.

The only reason for you to be wanting to smoke a cigarette or having an urge is purely psychological, it's imaginary, its face, it's not real! And because of all the previous mentioned descriptions, you should not smoke.

You need to retrain and re-educate yourself to go through beautiful life without smoking, and you can do it, you 've done it for the last two weeks now.

This is going to be a very tender and emotional period for you, stay the course and embrace your smoke-free status. You recognize how much better you are without smoking, clean clothes, no more yellow teeth and hands, your breath is smelling amazing, people don't cover their nose every time you talk to them. Your health level is better than when you were a smoker, you can do activities that were forbidden as a smoker, like walking, jogging, doing any kind of exercise you wish.

All those money you save now can be turned into anything you wish for, vacations, pick up a hobby, clothes, shoes, help a family member anything you want.

What should I call myself

I never thought of labeling myself after I quit smoking. I mean I was not smoking anymore.

A lot of people thought to feel the need to name their current status, and I see a lot of definitions online about how to describe someone that is not a smoker anymore.

Some say I am a non-smoker others say I am a former smoker others say they are ex-smokers which if you take them grammatically they are all correct give a take.

I didn't pay much attention to the need of labeling myself until I started reading three books about smoking (Allen Carr's The Only Way to Stop Smoking Permanently Joel Spitzer;s Never Take Another Puff and John R. Polito's Freedom from Nicotine – The Journey Home). They all address an issue that I didn't think about but I recognize some minor similarities in my behavior lately, and I want to discuss them here too.

The problems I encountered were two events that made me panic a little bit, to be honest.

One incident was at work there was a scene where some people were talking about going out and having a drink and just hearing them talk and describe the place they indented to go gave me this split second urge to pick up a cig and light it. The reason that happened was that I didn't deal with that scenario in real life without smoking because when I was a smoker every time I was going out for a drink, I would also smoke at the same time.

The other incident was similar to nature I was in the car, and I got jammed in traffic, and nothing was moving. At that split of second occurrences, I had that urge for a cigarette again something that made me panic again because I am smoke-free since 2009 there is no physiological reason to want to smoke.

These three books really helped me understand what is going with me and me now its must to name myself as an ex-smoker or a former smoker instead of a non-smoker because a non-smoker is someone that never smoked in his life ever.

It's important to relate this definition in my head because like it or not it reminds me that I was a drug addict and that I am a drug addict in recovery for the rest of my life. Like I said I might not like the sound of that but it's the truth and by me remind me that, the moments like I described before are not making me panic anymore because I know their origin.

I feel so much better since I quit smoking

Two months after I stop smoking me and my best friend went and visited Prague for a week, and it was the best time of my life because, except the beauty of the city itself I was on edge, I was feeling great, I had all this energy coming from seemingly nowhere.

All of this, of course, was because I stop killing myself with nicotine, carbon monoxide and another 4000 chemicals that are in the tobacco plant. About 60 to 80 of those chemicals are carcinogen which means they will give you cancer if you continue inhaling them into your body.

My smell started to coming back and oh my goodness I think we dined and had launched more than a dozen different restaurants in Prague I wanted to taste everything, my sense of smell also came back. I could detect aromas from a mile away and the most important of all I could smell tobacco from miles away and it was bothering me a lot, and that was a first indication that physiologically anyway I managed to get rid of smoking.

It was the first vacation I had in years without smoking, and I had a lot of challenges ahead of me, we drunk coffee and also beers, and also we ate a lot of food all those activities they were always accompanied by smoking.

To make it even worse, my friend was a smoker, so he smoked in front of me, but somehow I managed not to light one because I was determined that I was done with smoking.

Also, we must have visited half a dozen towers in Prague, the city is full of them, towers and clocks, I used the stairs to go to the top in all of them, and I felt great.

The fact that 2 months ago I couldn't walk ten steps without breathing like an old horse waiting to die and now I could go up 200 steps in one go was surprising.

My friend if there were not an elevator he would stay on the ground waiting for me and guess what he did, yep he smoked.

What I didn't know back then and of course now I know because of all the research I did for the book you are reading is this. I felt great because I was not smoking that's how good feels, that's how ordinary people that do not smoke are!

But for me to be able to do all those things felt like I suddenly acquired superman powers.

Now I realized how under the drug I was, how Nicotine and all the rest 3999 chemicals of tobacco crippled my body but most important took my mental, psychological and emotional freedom away from me.

Now that I ran marathons I feel great because let's face it not all people ran marathons as a hobby!

Another reason I wrote this book is that I don't want to forget that I was a smoker, that's how many ex-smokers return to smoking. They don't remember how bad it was, I wrote this book so it will be a constant reminder that I was a smoker and I don't want to do anything that will throw me back to the nicotine trap and prison, I am finished with that life forever. My only hope is that you are finished with the nicotine addiction also.

Have a healthy and Happy day, every day.

My Warmest Regards,

Andreas Michaelides

Other books by Andreas Michaelides

16 Common Smoking Rationalizations Recognized, Analyzed And Ultimate Destroyed.

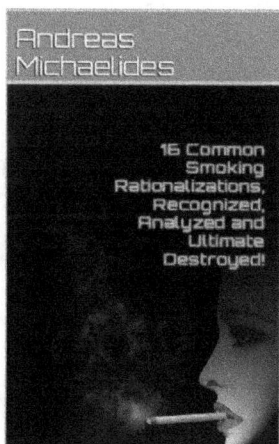

My fellow people, non-smokers, ex-smokers, and current smokers, let's begin the catharsis, let's learn a few useful truths of what smoking is, what nicotine is, and arm ourselves with some solid truthful, factual arguments to use. The non-smokers and ex-smokers can use them when they talk with other smokers and for the smokers to help them come to that realization point that you are a drug addict, and you need to recover to your previous nicotine free state, because trust me, that state is where you will find your true self.

How Not to Gain Weight After Quitting Smoking

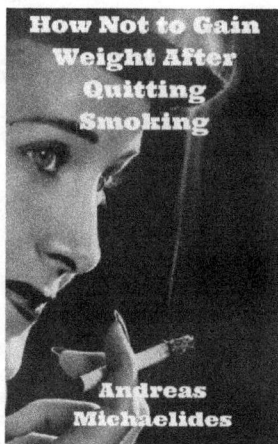

You think the governments increase the price of cigs and add more taxes because they want to help smokers quit? Hell no, they know they are dealing with an addiction. A smoker will pay anything to get their fix. When I was a smoker, and it happened to be 2 a.m., all hell broke loose if I was out of cigs. I would walk kilometers to find a kiosk open to buy cigs. Nothing stopped me from getting my fix!

Write a review.

I consider myself as a person that wants to think that I am continually improving my books, my work and myself. I am always trying to deliver to my readers the best quality and current information out there as my area of interest and expertise is a concern which is Health, Nutrition, and Exercise.

To accomplish that I need feedback from you and the only feedback I know that will help me achieve a relative perfection in all areas of my life is your valuable reviews, so I know where I am wrong or where I have made mistakes and errors.

There is no such thing as a perfect book out there, perfection for one person is a sloppy work for other, so to satisfy as much as people out there my books need to be regularly updated and it doesn't matter if it is in electronic form (Kindle) or paperback form.

If you found this book useful, please leave your review with all your thoughts, don't hold back, it will only take a few minutes of your time.

If you didn't like this book, please let me know by contacting me, and I will give my best shot to fix the issue.

Thank you very much,

My warmest regards

Andreas Michaelides